To Bill –

With love,

11/7/97   Elaine

THE BEST
I CAN

Odyssey of a Survivor

by

Elaine Phelps

FACTOR PRESS

Copyright © 1998 by Elaine Phelps
All rights are reserved.
No part of this book may be reproduced by any means,
electronic or mechanical, including photocopying without
permission in writing from the author, except in reviews.

Publisher's Cataloging-in-Publication Data
Phelps, Elaine.
The best I can: odyssey of a survivor / Elaine Phelps
p.cm.
ISBN 1-887650-09-1
1. Phelps, Ross - Biography. 2. Cancer-Patients-Biography.
3. Osteosarcoma. 4. Caregivers. 5. Chemotherapy.
I. National Institutes of Health. II. National Cancer Institute.
III. Title.
RC280.B6P54 1968

Jacket Illustration
Karmen Heflin Askew, Saratoga, California

Graphic Design
Fairhope Creative, Fairhope, Alabama

PUBLISHED IN THE UNITED STATES OF AMERICA

Factor Press
P.O. Box 8888
Mobile, AL 36689

In memory of my two sisters,
Hilda Heflin and Dorothy Riorda.

To my two sisters,
Vilma Croom and Jean Persons, and,

to Bill,

to Mary,

to Scott,

and

to Ross,

with love, and prayers.

Acknowledgments

Thank you long-time loyal supportive friends who have read, encouraged, critiqued, suggested, advised, and edited: Sally Green, Helen Meador, Zaidee Galloney, and Rosemary Fittje.

Thank you Karmen Heflin Askew, my niece and my friend, for listening to hours of discussion about the project, for sharing her talents in the jacket illustration and for believing in me.

My grateful appreciation to Robert Bahr, editor and publisher of Factor Press, for sharing his friendship, expertise, and generosity. Thanks also, to the talented and conscientious Ray Redlich, Graphics Designer, for his contribution and his patience.

And to all of you, from many of these United States and several foreign countries, who have touched Ross's life with hope and brought forth courage, I thank you.

Author's note:
This is a true story; however, many names have been changed to protect privacy.

THE BEST
I CAN

Odyssey of a Survivor

Prologue

September, 1982

He sat on a plastic modular chair, his eyes darting from child to child in the crowded waiting room. His 10:00 a.m. appointment obviously had been given to many others because each time the elevator door opened, another group of patients and their families filed in. An attractive teenaged girl entered on crutches, and Ross rose from his seat with only a quick glance at the space where her leg once was.

He walked over to a book rack on the wall and selected a brochure. After scanning a few pages, he wrinkled his brow, ran his fingers through his dark red hair, and quickly put the pamphlet back in its place. With shoulders slumped, he stared at the floor.

Towering over the youngsters playing on the floor, he picked his way around wheelchairs and toys, and walked over to where I stood near the window. His haunted eyes focused on my face; his skin paled. He quietly called to me, "Mom?"

"What, Ross?" I asked.

"I don't think you should read any of those brochures." His eyes widened, and he slowly shook his head. "Are you sure we're in the right place? There's mostly little kids in here."

"We're in the right place—the Pediatric Oncology Clinic."

"What does that mean—pediatric oncology?"

"I guess we'll soon find out," I whispered. I turned from him and stared out the floor-to-ceiling windows of the Clinical Center of the National Cancer Institute in Bethesda, Maryland. Thirteen floors below, I gazed at a sea of dark green trees slowly rippling in the early autumn breeze.

Ross stood beside me. His agile, athletic body maintained near-perfect posture for his five-foot eight-inch 145-pound frame. In a few days, he would be 18 years old. His skin, sprinkled with freckles, and his dark red hair had been his nemesis throughout childhood and adolescence, but finally he had made peace with it.

Across the waiting room near the door, Ross's father stood leaning his back against the wall, his arms folded and his shoulders rounded as if weighted down by a heavy load. Gray streaks shone in his light brown hair and neatly trimmed beard. Staring at some distant space, looking neither left nor right, his blue eyes were impenetrable.

Ross's older sister and brother, Mary and Scott, had been sitting rigidly on a sofa next to a rocking horse and pedal car, their eyes scanning around the room. As the room became crowded, Scott unfolded his lanky frame, rose from the couch, and walked over to stand by his dad, his dark brown eyes searching the room until he found me. Almost 20 years old, he was to begin college classes in a week.

Mary had taken the day off from her job on Capitol Hill where she worked for one of Alabama's senators. Twenty-six years old, her sense of adventure had always been a bellwether for Scott and Ross. Usually confident, assertive, and sophisticated, she met no strangers, but today she was quiet. When she turned to look at me, her dark eyes were liquid, and her lips were fixed in a tense smile. Her mane of black hair glistened to match the sparkle in her eyes. At five-feet three inches tall, she was the shortest member of the family, but her presence made up the difference.

My three children had one thing in common: dark brown, inscrutable eyes with which they communicated with each other.

Silently, Ross and I stood looking out the window at the leaves swaying gently in the wind far below. A few modern buildings dotted the forest miles away. A jet sparkled in the sun as it made its approach to Washington National Airport. In the distance, a white church steeple rose above the trees.

I turned when I heard a voice call out, "Ross Phelps?"

Ross followed the attendant along the hall. He walked with purpose, with confidence, and without any obvious nervousness—a young recruit reporting for an unknown assignment. Overhead lights along the hall revealed the sun streaks in his hair.

As my eyes followed him, I recalled the baby with fine wisps of red hair, the incessantly inquisitive toddler who marveled at simple things, the energetic little boy who loved and accepted love with joy. And the mischievous adolescent, the creative thinker, his antennae picking up all stimuli. Yet he had developed a steely control, and was labeled by his friends as "cool" and "laid back."

As Ross and the attendant disappeared around a corner at the end of the hall, I turned again to the window. The sea of green trees was just a blur.

So full of life, Ross was a senior in high school—confident in his ability to make many friendships. He was proud to be goalie on his high school soccer team, worked hard at his studies, and played harder—always in a hurry to do whatever it is that teenagers find so urgent.

Was it a month ago when he first mentioned that his wrist hurt? Or two months? I'd thought he'd said, "wrists"—both wrists. Since he'd had a summer job in a warehouse stacking heavy cases of beverages, I paid scant attention to his complaints.

Until the day he stayed home alone on Labor Day instead of going to the beach with friends. When Bill and I walked into the house in the late afternoon, we found him waiting for us. He solemnly announced, "I have to see a doctor about my wrist."

And the next day when he went to see an orthopaedic surgeon...

And the following morning, when Bill and I met with the doctors....

Another voice called out, "Mrs. Phelps?"

I turned from the window and held up my hand.

A young man wearing a starched white coat said, "I'm Dr. Raynor of the surgery staff. Will you come with me please?"

Bearded, wearing horn-rimmed glasses, he stood tall in wooden clogs and argyle socks.

As we walked together, he turned to me and said, "Dr. Sugarbaker and I have just told Ross that his condition appears to be osteosarcoma. If a biopsy confirms this, his left arm will have to be amputated."

I slowed my steps to a stop, then breathed deeply. "You've already told him about the amputation?" I whispered.

Dr. Raynor looked down at the floor, then lifted his eyes to mine. "Yes. It's best this way."

PART ONE

September, 1982—December, 1983

1

Ross sat on a straight-back wooden chair in the tiny examination room. His head and shoulders were to his knees. A young man, wearing a long white hospital coat, sat next to him, leaning forward, with his arm around Ross's shoulder.

"This is Dr. Paul Sugarbaker, Mrs. Phelps," Dr. Raynor said.

Dr. Sugarbaker rose and took my hand in his. He brushed his sandy-colored, curly hair from his forehead, and his clear blue eyes looked directly at me when he said, "We have just explained to Ross that his X-rays and examination indicate osteosarcoma—bone cancer. We're scheduling a biopsy, and if our suspicions are correct, his left arm will have to be amputated."

Ross was frozen, staring at the floor.

The surgeons quietly eased out of the room and closed the door, each one reaching to touch my shoulder as they passed.

Ross began to moan in short, shallow sobs. He turned his head and looked up at me with terror. "Now I understand," he whispered. "I know why you've been upset. I'm sorry, I didn't understand."

"...You're going to be all right..."

He stood up and fell against me, clutching my shoulders.

"You have to call the shots, Ross," I stammered. "Whatever you decide, is okay with me. You're not alone..."

We were interrupted by the first of several groups of doctors who rushed into the room, looked at the X-rays, examined Ross's wrist, and asked a barrage of questions.

"Have you ever taken steroids?" someone asked.

"No," said Ross.

"Yes," I said. "Remember when you had that rash on your feet a couple of years ago? You took a steroid drug then."

"He's talking about *steroids*, Mom. You know? Body-building steroids?"

When that group left, another man came strolling in alone. Over six feet tall, he wore a spotless white hospital coat, shiny shoes, and had black, slicked-down hair. He lifted the X-ray we had brought from Mobile and held it up to the light. He seemed unaware that we were in the room.

"I'm Elaine Phelps. This is my son, Ross."

"I'm Doctor Bradley Cook," he said, without looking at us.

"Have you seen the pediatrician's report I brought from Mobile?" I asked.

"I saw it," he said, shrugging his shoulders.

"Was it helpful?"

"It contributes nothing." He turned, glanced at me and said, "I am a surgeon, Mrs. Phelps. We know what we're doing. We don't require an old record from a pediatrician to make a diagnosis." He started out the door.

"Please wait," I said. "There's a lot I can tell you about his history. Wouldn't that be helpful?" I wanted to tell someone of Ross's digestive problems when he was a baby and that he had been unable to tolerate milk products. In infancy and early childhood he drank apple juice, and I worried about calcium deficiencies. I wanted somebody to acknowledge that this problem could be something else. "Could this have something to do with porous bones? He's had a broken bone in each foot. He plays soccer. Could it be fragile bones?"

The doctor rocked back and forth on his heels, his eyes darting around the room, and said, "Not likely."

Ross had turned his back to the door and faced the wall, but when another group of doctors jammed into the room, he whirled around, searching their faces, watching for a response when they looked at the X-rays. Some of the doctors hurried in, took a look, and walked out. Others looked closely at Ross's wrists and at the X-rays.

Everything was moving too fast. I said to anyone who would look at me, "Ross's eating habits aren't good...He drinks far too many carbonated drinks. And he started a high-dosage vitamin routine that's worried me...He doesn't get enough rest...."

They quietly nodded their heads as I babbled on, but it was obvious that they were not hearing anything I said. What might be a contributing cause was not important now.

Dr. Raynor returned to the room carrying a clipboard. "I have you set up, Ross. Here's your schedule for tests and scans. Note the time for the injection in preparation for the bone scan is eight-thirty tomorrow morning. After your tests are finished on Friday, you're free until Sunday afternoon when you have to be admitted no later than one o'clock for the biopsy on Monday morning."

"This coming Monday?" I asked.

"Yes. This cannot be delayed. The receptionist will tell you where to report tomorrow morning. I'll see you on Sunday after-noon, Ross."

Ross sat back down in the chair, folded his arms on the exam-ination table and leaned his head forward, shielding his eyes. "How long have you known about this, Mom?"

"A week."

"Does Dad know?"

"Yes."

"And Mary and Scott?"

"Mary does. Scott doesn't."

"Did Dr. King tell you?"

"He and Dr. Daugherty. Dr. Taylor agreed."

"Why didn't you tell me?"

"I didn't believe them."

"But you believe them now?" he asked. His shoulders started shaking and sobs quietly spilled out.

"No, no, I don't—not until more tests are done. They could be wrong, Ross. All of them could be wrong."

After a few minutes, he stood up, wiped his eyes and said, "Let's get out of here!"

Bill, Mary, and Scott were watching for us, and, when they saw us coming along the hall, they followed us to the elevator. Bill turned his head away. Mary posed questions with her eyes. Scott stared at me.

Mary, our chauffeur, maneuvered through the traffic on Rockville Pike, then turned onto a winding street toward Linden Hills Hotel. Together, we rode silently in the elevator and entered our room. Ross went into the bathroom and closed the door. The others turned to me.

As I tried to tell what had happened in the examination room, Scott paled and walked out on the little balcony outside our 10th floor room.

The bathroom door opened, Ross walked out and said, "Can't you please go somewhere else to talk? I want to be alone."

As Scott whirled through the room and out the door, Bill said, "Let's go for a walk."

Mary and I followed and the four of us walked together around the hotel's spacious landscaped grounds. We separated and met again by the pool. We discussed the possibility of finding another treatment center in some other city, and getting other doctors' opinions. We cried.

Bill said, "We've looked all over the United States. Several doctors in Mobile have helped us try to find the best place. I see no point in flying around all over the country trying to find somebody who'll say it's not so."

Scott walked hurriedly down the path toward the street. Mary's face crumbled again. Bill's shoulders sagged a little lower as he wandered off alone.

After an hour, we met in the hotel lobby and entered the elevator. When we walked into our room, we saw Ross face-down on one of the king-sized beds. His pillow was wet. Bill sat down on the sofa and flipped through a magazine. Scott paced the floor and I walked out on the balcony.

Mary lay down on the bed next to Ross. She said, "I know this really neat place to go for dinner. Let's get out of here and do something besides stare at each other."

"Go ahead. I don't want to go," Ross mumbled through the pillow.

"Come on, Ross," Scott said. "We didn't have much lunch and I'm starved."

Mary kissed Ross on the cheek and said, "Come on. Let's wash your face."

"I don't need any help washing my face, Mary. Leave me alone. Where did you want to go?"

"Wait and see," she said. She took his hand and pulled him up from the pillow.

Since Mary had become familiar with the area on a scouting trip the day before, she drove us down Wisconsin Avenue to the restaurant. She and Scott kept up a constant, jittery babble, and sang along with the music on the radio.

"What was that guy's name, Ross?" asked Scott. "Studebaker or Shake'n Baker?"

Mary giggled, and she and Scott started a chant in time with the music, "Stu-de-baker, Shake-n-baker, Sug-ar-baker...."

They talked about the mobs of people at the hospital, the various nationalities and their manner of dress. Ross silently stared out of the window.

All five of us crowded into a booth in the dark, crowded restaurant. After looking at the menu, Ross made his choice. The Hamburger Hamlet's bill of fare listed their special for the day—a hamburger so large it "takes two hands to hold it."

The music was loud and the young customers shouted over it. When we finished eating, Scott and Mary put their arms around Ross and the three of them walked slowly to the parking lot ahead of us. The street lights shone down on them through a foggy, misty rain.

During the next day and a half, Ross endured a barrage of tests, X-rays, and CAT scans. We learned our way around the enormous Clinic Center building as the whole family followed him for what seemed like miles from one appointment to another.

On Saturday, Scott flew back to Mobile to attend to the family pets and prepare for school, and Mary went back to her apartment.

Bill, Ross, and I attended a folk mass on Sunday morning in the basement of the National Cathedral, then had brunch at a restaurant in Georgetown before returning to the hospital for Ross's admission.

The admitting procedure took hours. Many forms and permissions contracts had to be thoroughly examined before signing. Ross had reached his 18th birthday just the day before, and he signed the consent papers, but they asked me to co-sign.

We were directed to the 10th floor—the surgery wing—where we found the hall crowded with staff and equipment. Ross's roommate, an elderly man in great pain, was unaware when he carried his things to the windowed side of the room. The man cried out, begging for someone to help him. We had no idea that these would be his final hours.

Bill and I left when visiting hours were over. Later, I telephoned Ross from our hotel. "You okay?" I asked.

"I'm all right, I guess."

"How's your roommate? Has he gone to sleep?"

"No. But I've been out of the room a lot. I can't leave the floor, but I found a telephone watts line. I talked to Jim and Kit. I've been visiting with some other patients, and they told me about the phone."

"Will you call me if you need anything?"

"I'm okay, Mom. Quit worrying about me."

Early the next morning, Bill and I watched as he crawled over on the gurney and began his journey. The attendants stopped at the surgery hall door, just enough time for us to kiss Ross on his forehead.

He was given general anesthesia but the biopsy was quick. He was back in his room in two hours, but had not been forewarned about the intense pain he would experience.

The surgeons told us it would be several days before the report was complete because the samples taken had to go through a decalcification process before the final diagnosis.

That evening, the Tumor Board met for evaluation and discussion of new cases. The Board was composed of physicians from all over the United States and abroad.

Still groggy from anesthesia, Ross was taken by wheelchair to the conference room. He sat on the stage while his case was presented by Dr. Sugarbaker to Dr. Rosenberg, Chief of Surgery. Bill and I were barred from the conference, but observed the stage from a side door. We could see Ross's X-rays projected on a screen behind him and Dr. Rosenberg.

I couldn't hear what was being said, but understood that a well-known limb-sparing specialist was present and thought certain he would intervene against the planned amputation. The longer they discussed Ross's case, the more hopeful it seemed. A few doctors walked up on stage from the auditorium to look closer at the images. Dr. Sugarbaker seemed to be speaking about the biopsy. The limb-sparing specialist said nothing.

After the conference, I learned that the principal discussion centered on why there had been two separate incisions for removal of tissue samples. Dr. Sugarbaker explained that the first incision revealed a mass which was encapsulated and they chose not to break into the outer covering. They reentered at an alternate spot and found the mass had broken through, making the bone and tissue samples accessible.

The following day, Ross was discharged from the hospital and Bill returned to Mobile. On Wednesday, I flew home, leaving Mary as much in charge as Ross would permit. Mary was to be in a wedding in Mobile the following weekend, so together they flew home on Thursday. We were told that the doctors would call when the final pathology report was completed.

2

Back in Mobile, amid the chaos of unpacked and half-packed luggage, we found it impossible to return to our routine lives. Although our house had been a perfect size when the children were small, now five adults bumped into each other at bathroom doors or when reaching for car keys. Even our yard, with its giant oak trees, seemed too small.

The telephone rang constantly; visitors were in and out of the house. Ross's Aunt Vilma and Aunt Jean brought food and stood by waiting for instructions. Cars lined our driveway and the street out front, and neighbors slowed when driving or walking past.

Our neighborhood in the Spring Hill suburb of Mobile had begun almost 100 years before. As the area grew throughout the years, the houses that were built ranged from grand to modest. Our house fell into the second category, but its design was somewhat different from all the others. The rooms downstairs had a wall of glass, and each of the four bedrooms upstairs had a double sliding glass window which looked out over a patio shaded by oak, dogwood, and magnolia trees. Ivy tumbled over a high brick privacy wall.

The kitchen was our meeting place—our conference room— where important matters were discussed while sitting at a round white pedestal table surrounded by chairs with bright gold, red, or orange cushions. Although there were phones upstairs, the community telephone hung on the kitchen wall.

On Friday, the day of waiting, the tension was palpable, and each time the phone rang, everyone froze.

In the late afternoon, Dr. Raynor called. "Mrs. Phelps? Dr. Raynor at NIH. Tell Ross that the pathologist's report is positive. He must be here Tuesday for conferences. The surgery will be done on Thursday."

Ross studied my face and, without a word, he turned and went to the patio outside the kitchen door.

I repeated Dr. Raynor's words to Bill, then to Mary and Scott. I telephoned Vilma, and her husband, Joe Croom, who lived a couple of blocks away.

I discussed the whole situation with a friend who was a physician. He listened with compassion, and, somewhere in our conversation, he said, "You'll have to quit your job."

Six months earlier I had returned to full-time employment for the first time in many years. Bill's architectural work was in a slump, and we faced the prospect of having two sons in college at the same time. I was fortunate to get a good job with a well-known Mobile based corporation. However, without clearly understanding why it would be necessary that I give up the position, I followed my friend's advice and turned in my resignation with very little advance notice.

Ross moved around like a zombie. As the news spread, awe-struck teenage friends surrounded him. Their response, while sometimes overwhelming, kept him from despair.

When he was home alone with me, his emotions began to whirl, rise and fall. I invited him to use me as a sounding board—a decision I would question in the months to come.

The days following Dr. Raynor's call flew by. Bill decided we must have an automobile in Bethesda, so he and Mary left early Tuesday morning, driving my car to Birmingham where she would meet her boss and other staff members for a trade conference there. Bill would drive on to Bethesda. Scott would take charge of the house and the various pets while he worked his part-time job and attended school at the University of South Alabama.

Ross and I were to fly to Washington that same morning. I called to him from downstairs, "Ross, we have to hurry."

"I'll make it," he called back.

He didn't sound sleepy, and I wondered how long he had been awake. I couldn't hear him moving around so I went upstairs to get his luggage. He was sitting on the side of his bed, not dressed.

"Get moving, Ross. We have to leave in a few minutes."

"I'll be ready," he said, staring at the floor.

After I left him, I heard the shower running and wondered about logistics if we missed the plane. As I went down the stairs, I heard a knock on the door. Several of his classmates stood outside. They had skipped school in order to say good-bye. "Your timing is good," I said. "I could use some help."

They tramped noisily up the stairs. I could hear teasing, scuffling, and nervous laughter mixed with words of encouragement.

"Come on, man! Get with the program! Move, Phelps. Get the lead out! Go, man, go!"

In a few minutes, they escorted Ross down the stairs. "We'll drive him to the airport, Mrs. Phelps. Meet you there," they shouted. I could hear cars cranking up, racing their motors, and moving out in a caravan.

Checking our luggage and tickets at the airport, I walked rapidly through the almost deserted terminal. Just before going through the security gate to look for Ross, the clamorous contingent of boys arrived and ushered him to the departure gate where they mixed good-byes with yells of assurance.

On the plane, after fastening his seat belt, Ross adjusted the overhead light and air valve, pulled out all the pamphlets and magazines from the seat pocket, tapped his fingers, and fidgeted with everything in reach.

"When we get up there, Mom, I'll need your help. We won't have much time, and I don't think I can do it all by myself."

"Do what by yourself?"

"Find out the name of every doctor who was in the Tumor Board meeting. I want to talk to every one of them and find out what they have to say."

"I doubt you can do that. There were about fifty in there."

"We can try. I'll talk to some doctors and you talk to others."

"What questions do you want me to ask?"

"Find out what they think. See if they know of anyone who has had what I have in the same place and find out what happened to them. Ask if they had amputations or could they do something else. Find out if they know somewhere else I could go where they could try something different."

"Do you think we could get another conference?" I asked.

"I want to talk to that limb-sparing guy."

"I don't know about that. He's not on the staff of NIH."

"Find out, will you? Please, Mom. Help me."

"Okay. I don't know where to start. I'll ask for a conference as soon as we get there."

After making our connection in Atlanta, Ross settled down to watch the horizon from the airplane window. But as soon as the seat belt light went off, he rose and paced up and down the aisle. He asked for a cup of water and lingered at the station, talking with a flight attendant. He didn't eat a luncheon sandwich, but he drank water and Cokes. When we landed at Dulles Airport, he stood quickly and reached into the overhead compartment for his backpack.

Mary had left her car at the airport for us to use until Bill arrived with mine. Ross rushed me from the baggage claim through the parking lot. Then he got behind the wheel and drove onto the Beltway at high speed. As he pulled up in front of the Clinic Center, he said, "Go on up to the surgery clinic while I park the car. Ask for Dr. Sugarbaker. Tell him what I said."

"I'll ask if he will arrange a conference."

"Don't ask him, Mom. Tell him I want one now. Okay?"

When Ross joined me in the surgery clinic, I told him that all I had accomplished was to tell the receptionist that I wanted to see Dr. Sugarbaker. He whirled around and marched up to the desk. After a heated discussion, the receptionist pointed around the hall and he strode down and turned into an office. In a few minutes, he walked back to the waiting room.

"I saw him. He's fixing a conference for two o'clock. The

limb-sparing guy's name is Dr. Martin Malawer. He can't be there, but there'll be several other doctors."

"We'll have time to check into the hotel."

"I'm not leaving. I'm going to find some more doctors."

"Let's go to the cafeteria," I said, rising from my chair.

"No, I'm not leaving. You can bring me some iced tea."

At 2:00 p.m., in a small conference room, five surgeons sat around the table: Dr. Sugarbaker, Dr. Raynor, Dr. Cook, and two others whose names I couldn't recall. Ross sat at the end of the table; my chair was near the door.

"Thank you for coming," Dr. Sugarbaker said, as he nodded to his colleagues. "Ross has asked us to go over his case again." Turning to Ross, he asked, "Do you have specific questions, Ross?"

"I want to know what my options are," Ross said.

The doctors were silent, each with their eyes averted.

Dr. Sugarbaker opened the big brown envelope and pulled out the X-rays. "Come over here, Ross. Let's talk about this again." He rose and pushed his chair aside, then lifted the X-rays up to the light.

Ross walked over and stood beside him.

Pointing his finger at the film, Dr. Sugarbaker said, "You can see right here how all the bones are involved at the wrist. The entire area shows destruction."

"Can't you remove the tumor and parts of the bone?"

"No. See how it has advanced toward the elbow? Destruction is moving up the radius. The wrist offers no room to work. All the nerves and blood vessels which supply your hand—everything is confined into a very narrow space."

Ross looked at each one of the other doctors, then returned to his chair. "Can't you burn the tumor out with radiation?"

Dr. Raynor spoke up, "Ross, our evidence does not indicate that radiation is effective against osteosarcoma. Even if it was, you would have no further use of your arm and hand. They would be burned black."

"And you still wouldn't be sure you had accomplished anything regarding the spread of the disease," a young man added.

Ross rested his elbows on the table and rubbed his forehead.

"You're better off than a lot of our patients, Ross," Dr. Sugarbaker said. "We plan to measure six inches from the tumor, which will leave your elbow. You should have good use of the rest of your arm with a prosthesis."

Ross continued to keep his head down with his hand shielding his eyes. "Could I try the chemotherapy first and see if it does any good? Wouldn't it maybe kill the tumor and make it stop growing?"

"Chemotherapy acts against microscopic cancer cells, but it's not usually as effective against a tumor...."

"The bone is already destroyed in places...."

"It's a wonder your arm hasn't already broken...."

Ross straightened up and looked from face to face. "I think I should have some options. Can't you tell me what they are?"

Dr. Sugarbaker turned to him. "The only options you have are to do nothing at all, or agree to the amputation. If you choose to do nothing, your chances of living much longer are almost non-existent. If you don't agree to the amputation, there is nothing we can do for you. I'm sorry...I wish I had a better answer."

Dr. Sugarbaker stood and picked up the X-rays. One by one around the table, the others pushed their chairs back and started moving toward the door. They stopped and patted Ross's shoulder as they passed.

Ross continued to sit, his hands covering his face. I walked out into the hall, leaned my back against the wall, and watched the surgeons hurrying to their clinics and offices. In a few minutes, Ross came out into the hall and looked at me, searching.

I took his hand, squeezed it tightly, and said, "Do you want to go to the hotel now?"

"I want to talk to that guy who's saved limbs—Malawer."

"Let's find a phone," I said. "He's at George Washington University, or Georgetown, I think. Maybe he's at Children's Hospital."

We hurried back to the receptionist's desk and asked how to get in touch with Dr. Malawer. She said that it would be difficult to get an appointment with him on short notice.

Dr. Sugarbaker walked up as we were talking. "Dr. Malawer

can't do anything, Ross. There's no way to do a limb-sparing surgery in this confined area."

Tears shot forward in Ross's eyes. He turned his head and walked a few steps away.

"Is it possible to take some more X-rays?" I asked. "Maybe this thing has shrunk on its own."

"No, Mrs. Phelps," he said, shaking his head. "Ross, let me look at your wrist. See? If anything, the mass is getting larger."

I looked at Ross's wrist. He was right. It was larger.

On Wednesday, Ross was admitted to the 10th floor for surgery. His room, across the hall from the nurses' station, was occupied by a man who appeared to be about 35 years old. Dressed in jogging shorts, a tee shirt, athletic socks and shoes, he sat on the floor with his legs stretched out, bending forward to touch his toes. As we entered, he hopped up, reached out his hand to Ross, and said, "Come in, come in. I'm Bob McArthur."

"I'm Ross Phelps, and this is my mother."

"Where're you from?" he asked.

"Mobile, Alabama. How about you?"

"I live about ten miles from here—on the other side of Rockville."

"That must be great," I said. "It's a long trip from Mobile."

"It's nice because my wife can come to see me and bring whatever I need. If you need anything, let me know. She'll be glad to pick up stuff for you."

"Do you have the bed by the window?" Ross asked.

"Nope. It's all yours. I like the bed by the door."

Ross placed his backpack on a chair and stood looking out the window at the Bethesda skyline.

Bob stretched, ran in place for a few seconds, then sprinted down the hall and back.

"Are you training for a marathon?" I asked.

"No," he laughed. "Surgery. I'd rather do this than take

tranquilizers and sleeping pills. I know what to expect. I've been through a few operations. I'm better off if I'm in good shape."

"You've had surgery for cancer already?" asked Ross.

"More than once—several times. Pancreas. I hear you're to have your arm amputated."

"That's what they tell me. When are you scheduled?"

"The day after you, I think. I run up and down the hall rather than stay in bed and worry about it."

"This is new to us," I said. "It's pretty scary."

"You've got a right to be scared. But you've got to believe you can beat it. You've got to try. That's all I can do."

He walked over to the window and placed his arm around Ross's shoulder. "Ross, get your mind set. Get in the right frame of mind. It helps."

While on grand rounds, several surgeons witnessed Ross's signature on the consent form for the amputation. They must have known that I would rebel against signing it, because they didn't ask me. I went out into the hall and covered my face with my hands.

A doctor left Ross's room, hurried past me, and said, "Your son has just done one of the most bitter things a young man will ever have to do."

Another said, "Life isn't fair, Mrs. Phelps. Princess Grace died today in an automobile accident."

I wondered why he said that.

As the surgeons left, a procession of anesthesiologists, lab technicians, and occupational therapists entered Ross's room. One of the occupational therapists, a young lady named Bonnie, had big brown eyes, and she told him that her eyes would be the first thing he would see when he woke from the anesthesia. She said that after the surgery, she would put a cast on his arm.

I followed her out of the room and down the hall.

"You have a very angry son, Mrs. Phelps," Bonnie said, as she rolled her big brown eyes. "He's going to have to work his way through this."

"I don't know how," I said. "I'm angry, too."

"Your anger isn't helping him. Try to put some distance between the two of you. Let Ross deal with it in his own way."

"He's only eighteen. He's never faced anything like this."

"None of our patients have. It's devastating, but he'll be all right. We'll be working with him for a long, long time and get to know him very well. When we begin therapy, I want him free from damaging emotional entanglements. Let me remind you there are attitudes that can be just as crippling as the loss of a limb."

∾

Ross asked for a pass from the hospital for the evening. Bill had arrived, ending his long drive from Mobile, so we repeated our usual trek to Wisconsin Avenue, where we silently wandered among the crowd and went through the motions of having dinner. When we returned Ross to the 10th floor, we said goodnight, leaving him with his own thoughts.

Later, I learned that he again went to the watts line and called his best friend in Mobile, Jim Phillips, and said, "I've just signed my arm away."

Early the next morning, Bill and I accompanied the gurney on the long walk to the surgery hall door. Although Ross had been given premeds, his eyes were wide as he turned his head to look up at me.

While the entourage moved slowly, he asked, "Mom? Will you hold my hand?" His eyes brimmed as they focused on his uplifted left hand.

He gripped my hand with unusual strength as I leaned over to kiss him at the swinging double door. When the door closed, Bill and I slowly turned away and returned to the surgery waiting room. I signed out with the receptionist and left to get out of the building.

Dark clouds whirled overhead as I walked the grounds, still begging God to intervene. I stopped and stared at bright lights in what I thought were the windows of the surgery theater. I wondered what would happen if lightning caused a power failure. Big drops of rain began to fall.

When I returned to the waiting room, I saw the therapists, Bonnie, and her associate, walking along the hall. It must be almost time for their part of the procedure.

After uncounted minutes—maybe hours—Dr. Sugarbaker and Dr. Raynor came out to tell us the operation was over. They spoke softly in clinical terms that we could understand. Their eyes seemed weary and sad.

Shortly afterward, Ross was returned to his room with several attendants. He was beginning to come out of the anesthesia. A sheet and blanket covered him. There was an absence of form on his left side.

I sat beside the bed and waited.

He drifted in and out of consciousness, slowly becoming aware. He tried to speak, to say something. I couldn't understand, so I bent closer to his face.

"What do you want, Ross? Can I get you anything? Try to go back to sleep," I whispered.

"Go on, Mom...hurry," he mumbled.

"Where? What for?" I asked, as he drifted away again.

A few minutes later, he said, "Lab. The lab...hurry, Mom."

"The lab? Why, honey, why?"

"Find my arm. See what they're doing with my arm. I want to know what they're going to do with it."

I waited as he slipped away again.

Later, he turned his head and glared at me. "What time is it? Did you go to the lab? Did they say if it's in my blood stream?" His eyelids slowly closed again as he drifted back into his nightmarish world.

Opening his eyes widely, he asked, "Have you seen it?" He glanced at the large lump under the covers on his left side.

"No," I said.

"Don't touch it," he whispered, slowly closing his eyes.

When he became more fully awake and asked again if I had seen it, I said, "I will if you want me to."

Hesitating, he said, "Yes." He turned his head away.

I carefully lifted the covers. I saw a large, somewhat round, white plaster cast around his elbow, and nothing below it.

"What does it look like? What do you see?"

"...I see...I see that the cancer is gone."

From the other side of the curtained partition, Bob McArthur said, "That is an excellent description of the circumstances. Keep it in mind. It's gone."

Ross slowly turned his head and looked at his arm. His face crumpled and he appeared to be choking.

I kissed his cheek. "You are loved so much by so many people and this isn't going to make any difference. You'll still be loved—even more."

"I love everybody...will you tell them?" He was sobbing.

"I'll tell them. Go back to sleep."

As he became more wakeful, the intensity of his physical pain increased. He had the first of many experiences with "phantom" pain. Severe, twisting cramps in the absent hand and arm created a new dimension of reality.

Doctor Raynor stopped by. He explained that the nerve endings on the stump of the arm continued to send messages to the brain telling of trauma to the limb as though it was still attached. "Injury, surgery, or disease in the bone are among the most exquisite pains known," he said.

"Can't you do anything about it?" I asked.

"Not much, but it will get better," he said. "Ross, look up at the ceiling, lift your arms, then place your right hand on the spot where you feel the pain in your left hand."

Ross looked at him, then moved his eyes upward. He lifted his left arm, then moved his right hand to approximately where the left hand should be. "That's weird...it feels like it's still there."

"It's normal," the doctor said. "As days and weeks go by, I'll ask you to do this again. You'll find that the left hand sensation will gradually move nearer to the stump of your arm."

"Will it eventually disappear?" Ross asked.

"Not completely for a long time. But before long, it will feel as though your fingers are attached to the stump."

"When will the cramps go away?" Ross asked, as he grimaced in a new assault of pain.

"That's hard to say exactly, Ross. You'll continue to have them as long as the nerve endings are active. The only way to stop the pain is to kill the nerves in the stump, but we don't want to do that."

Bill quietly entered the room. His bearded face made it difficult to decipher his feelings. Although a couple of inches taller than I, he seemed now about the same height, as if he had withered. Even his chest seemed sunken, as though it had caved in. His lips were tightly drawn, his eyes vacant. Without speaking, he turned and left the room.

As the day drew to a close, Mary arrived, having been delivered to the front of the building by an army vehicle following an inspection trip she had been on with the senator and other staffers. When I stepped out into the hall, I saw her leaning against the wall with her hands covering her face. Her shoulders were shaking. A nurse handed her a cup of water.

"Please tell me they didn't have to amputate," she whispered. She clung to me and we silently cried together.

I lifted her hair from her forehead and whispered, "Are you all right? Can you go in now?"

She blew her nose, wiped her eyes, and entered the room. She said nothing as she leaned over the bed and kissed Ross, her tears falling on his face.

The phone rang and Bill answered it. He turned to face the window as he talked to Scott, trying to assure him that Ross would be all right.

Visiting hours were strictly enforced, and as Bill, Mary, and I were going down on the elevator, we talked of how cruel it seemed to leave Ross alone. Bill stared at the floor; Mary's eyes were swimming in tears. In our lives, there had been no other experience to compare with the pain of this day.

But an ominous scene unfolded when the elevator car stopped on the sixth floor and an attractive lady stepped on. Standing there at the door was a little child holding onto her IV pole. She had no hair, and only one arm.

"I love you, baby. Have a good night," the dry-eyed mother said.

"Goodnight, Mommy. See you in the morning," the child answered as the elevator door closed.

∾

October, 1982

Ross's days in the hospital bed after surgery were a mixture of intense pain, extreme nervousness, hyper-activity, and incessant talk. As his mind cleared from the pain medication, he kept up a constant chatter.

"As soon as I get home, I'm going to take flying lessons."

"Flying lessons? As in flying a plane?"

"Yes. There's no reason why I can't learn to fly."

"Let's wait and see...."

"I'm not waiting. I'm going to do it. Then I'm going to take parachuting. I can learn to do that, too. And maybe I can hang-glide. I've always wanted to sail through the air and let the wind currents take me."

"Ross..."

"Don't start discouraging me, Mom. Stop being so negative."

"I'm not being negative."

"Go look in the mirror. Look at the expression on your face. I don't need you to get in my way."

"You've never said anything about these things before."

"That's not all. I'm going to ask my friends' fathers if I can go with them on hunting trips."

"Hunting? You couldn't kill an animal or a bird."

"I've always wanted to go on a hunting trip. Dad's not interested, but I'd like to go. I'm going to learn to shoot a gun."

"There's a shooting range in Mobile. You could learn to shoot targets."

"Maybe, but I still want to go into the woods with a gun. I could practice on some tin cans."

"Okay."

"I've got to get out of here. There's so much I want to do. I'm not staying in this bed. There's no reason..."

"Let me ask the nurse," I said.

She came walking in and said, "I heard that, Ross. You can get out of the room in a wheelchair. No more walking to the watts line phone until your doctor says it's okay."

"A wheelchair! That's stupid! I can walk just fine."

"It may be stupid, but it's your ticket out of the room," the nurse said. "And your mom has to push the chair. No stretching or straining, okay?"

As I tried to get the chair in position and understand the mechanisms, Ross said, "We've got to have an understanding. You go where I tell you, when I tell you. Okay?"

"Suits me. Fasten your seat belt."

"I want to go to the downstairs lobby."

"Let me ask the nurses if we can leave the floor."

"Don't ask them. Tell them. I'm going wherever I want to go."

In the lobby, we maneuvered through the gallery toward the front entrance. Two policemen sat at the security station.

"Think I could be a cop?"

"I don't care what you do."

"I'm going to join the army."

"Ross, that's enough. Let's stop this talk for now."

"I'm going to the recruiting office and they're going to tell me I can't join. Then I'm going to sue them for discrimination. I'm going to do it."

"Okay, okay. The army can teach you how to shoot a gun."

"I have to learn how to shoot. I've got to learn how to defend myself...."

Bill flew back to Mobile on Monday, and Ross was discharged to the hotel Tuesday, continuing his heavy pain medication.

But it didn't matter. We had all been crawling out of a deep dark pit, and now the path seemed a little clearer. The cancer was gone.

3

But the doctors were not certain. Ross's first NIH social worker, Andy Tartler, joined us in the sixth-floor conference room where we met with the surgeons and oncologists. A warm and personable man in his middle thirties, Andy immediately established a close rapport with Ross. He quickly confirmed in Ross's mind that he was an ally—one who would be with him to walk through the maze of this new world.

Again, we sat around the conference table, Andy taking his position beside Ross. Andy wore a white shirt and tie, but removed his coat and rolled up his shirt sleeves. He placed his arm around the back of Ross's chair as they faced the doctors.

"What are my chances now?" Ross asked.

"There's no way to answer that question. Your chances may have improved," said Dr. Cook of the surgery staff. "You might have a better chance of beating the odds," he added, as he again quoted the grim statistics of survival with osteosarcoma.

"It doesn't sound very encouraging," Ross said.

"It's all we have to go on, Ross," Dr. Sugarbaker said. "We can only say that you have a fifty-fifty chance. You have the very big advantage of having no metastases that we can find. Many of our patients don't get to NIH until it's too late to do an amputation. Keep that in mind."

"But what can I do? What will help me?" Ross asked. "Will I

still get a metastasis? Can't you tell if it's in my bloodstream? Can't something be done?"

A weary-looking young man shook his head and said, "We don't know, Ross. We don't know any more about the cause, the spread, or the treatment of cancer than you do."

"Now wait a minute, doctor," Andy said, as he leaned forward. "That is not a very comforting thought. Not at all."

"It's the truth."

"Well, let's see if we can't give a little more thought to this and meet again tomorrow. Come on, Ross—Mrs. Phelps. Let's go to the cafeteria."

As we walked to the elevator, Andy said, "I'm sorry, Ross. I can't believe he said that. He must have had a bad day. Forget it. There are other things for you to consider."

The next day we again met for questions and answers. Percentages were tossed about as if they were supposed to mean something. It appeared that no one knew if the surgery really made any difference. Although the available facts were repeated, the whole picture was not in focus. No one said Ross's chances for recovery were excellent—or even good. They did not say it because they did not know.

Over and over in my mind, I said, Today is the only time anyone has...The present moment is all...Ross's chances are as good as anyone else's. We tried to believe that.

There was no test to determine if there were any malignant cells anywhere in Ross's body. If cancer cells were present somewhere, chemotherapy might be effective in destroying them while in their microscopic stage. The oncologists discussed their current studies, or clinical trials as they are called, and presented the option of participating to Ross.

One of the oncologists said, "Ross, if you want to consider chemotherapy, you'll have to allow us to place your name in the computer for random selection. One half of the group will start the protocol after definitive surgery. The other half will get no further treatment. We are trying to learn if the combination of these particular drugs are effective in treating osteosarcoma, thereby prolonging life."

"What do you mean, 'prolonging life'?" I asked. "Is there a

study anywhere that's investigating more than prolonging life—like maybe an outright cure?"

"We have hopes for all our studies, Mrs. Phelps. The word 'cure' is yet a ways off."

"Can you tell me of any other treatment centers that have anything promising?" Ross asked.

"No more than we have. Remember, it takes years to collect reliable data. We're aware of everything going on all over the country and in some foreign countries. We keep on top of it."

Another oncologist spoke up and said, "Ross, while we're on this subject, be careful not to believe rumors you hear about miracle cures. There are none. Don't let anybody use you and your condition. There are people in the world who will try to take advantage of your situation. Don't believe them. They're peddling false hope—and often making a lot of money on it. Just don't believe it."

"Another important consideration, Ross—and Mrs. Phelps," Andy began. "If you agree to participate, the treatment will be free of financial cost. You will be followed every step of the way by the staff here, including all departments, and your case will become part of the historical records."

We learned that the cost of chemotherapy treatment can be phenomenal. Unless one is very wealthy or has excellent insurance coverage, treatment for this type of cancer could be prohibitive. Ross's health insurance would be only a tiny drop in a deep well. When Andy had said, "free of financial cost," a glimmer of relief was born.

Because osteosarcoma is such a rare disease, it is difficult to find enough evidence to conduct a study. Since it is discovered at widely varying stages of development, and because no two patients react the same way to treatment, it seemed to be an impossible undertaking.

"Do you need to think about this, Ross? We can give you a day or two," Andy asked.

"No, I guess not," Ross said. "I don't see that I have any choice. I've got to do something, whatever there is I can do."

His name was placed in the study for random, computerized selection.

While waiting for the assignment process and while still recuperating from the amputation, we remained in the hotel with many trips back and forth to the busy NIH Occupational and Physical Therapy Department and to the school.

Since Ross had just begun his senior year in high school, he learned that, if he was selected for chemotherapy treatment, he could continue his studies in the hospital, where a school had been established by the Montgomery County, Maryland, Board of Education. Lessons could be taught at bedside when a patient was unable to go to the classroom in the Clinic Center.

We learned that the school occupies a very small area of the huge complex. The National Institutes of Health are situated on a 300-acre campus and maintains a 500-bed hospital. It employs more than 10,000 people, including hundreds of foreign scientists. There are 11 different Institutes, each devoted to a particular area of disease or disorder. It has more than 1,400 laboratories.

The Bethesda Naval Hospital, where many Presidents have received treatment, is across busy Rockville Pike, adjacent to the NIH campus. Walter Reed Army Hospital is about four miles away. Many private ancillary facilities are also close by.

In addition to the many laboratories on the NIH campus, the scientists have oversight in research in many universities, government facilities, and private laboratories throughout the United States. The yearly budget is several billion dollars.

It is one of the largest research centers in the world and houses the world's largest reference center at the National Library of Medicine.

Except for certain administrative offices and labs, no place is considered off-limits at NIH and we explored many areas of the Clinic Center and campus.

The Clinic Center is the hub of patient activity. Patients with almost every disorder known, or unknown, are seen there. The four aged elevators in the older part of the hospital are operator-assisted at times. All of them are on call for emergencies, which means getting off whenever asked. One elevator is usually in service for patient meals. Often, another is conscripted for moving furniture and building materials for the continuous on-going construction and remodeling. Most of the time, one elevator is out of order. The remaining car is invariably packed, and a long wait is necessary.

The upper floors of the Clinic Center are devoted to standard hospital patient rooms. There are a few scattered business offices and numerous labs. Each floor has four wings, one of which joins the newer addition, where the out-patient clinic is located.

We learned what conditions are given the name, "cancer." In the Pediatric Branch of the National Cancer Institute, only six different kinds of cancer were being treated: osteosarcoma, Ewing's sarcoma, neuroblastoma, rhabdomyosarcoma, non-Hodgkins lymphoma, and leukemia. These unfamiliar words, usually shortened in conversations, were often heard in the Clinic Center.

Only about 500 new cases of osteosarcoma are reported each year. Ewing's sarcoma, another form of bone cancer, is considered even more rare, with only about 250 new cases reported yearly.

Since there are more than 100 different types of cancer, I had to cut the definition down to a size I could grasp, knowing that it probably had little basis in scientific fact:

The cells in our bodies continually replace themselves by dividing and separating in an orderly way. There is a "control" in our system which, at the proper time, stops the cells from dividing. This control may be linked to our immune system or our genetic makeup. In a malignancy, the controlling function fails to stop the continuing division and multiplication of cells. The new cells, though weak and "confused," continue to increase until they become invasive to the tissue, organs, and bones surrounding them, destroying all in their path. Also, the malignant cells often break off, get into the blood stream, and form new colonies in various parts of the body, usually with some consistency, depending on the type of tumor involved.

In osteosarcoma, metastases are usually discovered first in the lungs. Sometimes they are found when the original site is discovered. I remembered Ross's consternation when the doctors in Mobile made an X-ray of his chest when his complaint was that his wrist hurt.

Lung metastases are not uncommon and are removed surgically. Often a patient has lung surgeries during the first two years of diagnosis. Patients call this procedure, "thoracotomy," and surgeons sometimes jokingly refer to it as "picking grapes."

The question as to whether or not metastases also metastasize was not clarified. Metastases continue to grow larger and perhaps spawn other nodules, which threaten and destroy other tissue and organs surrounding them.

Considering the complexity of the disease and the many forms it can take, this elementary definition sufficed and my understanding of cancer never progressed beyond that point.

Ross's agreement to participate in the study included therapy and teaching of ways to overcome some of the problems of the amputee. For him, the staff of the Physical and Occupational Therapy Departments were some of the most important in the entire facility. They gave Ross encouragement and confidence that he couldn't find elsewhere. They helped him to feel whole, in spite of the amputation.

The receptionist in Occupational Therapy called Ross at the hotel and asked him to come in to meet another patient who had also lost an arm to cancer two years before.

Patrick met Ross at a picnic table on the grounds outside the cafeteria. He appeared to be about Ross's age. He spoke with quiet confidence and immediately put Ross at ease. He told a little about himself—that he lived in Arizona with his mother and was in town to have his check-up and visit his father. He invited Ross to ask any questions about the use of the prosthesis.

"Do people stare at you?" Ross asked.

"Sure—sometimes. Especially the little kids. Everybody does, actually. At least, it seems they do. But it doesn't bother me much anymore. I guess I would stare, too."

Ross asked him about using the prosthesis for driving. Patrick explained that the device would be dangerous for driving and he would have to learn to drive with one hand.

After having left them alone for an hour, I returned to the picnic table in time to hear Patrick say, "One more thing, Ross. The most important thing to remember is that you are not handicapped. You only have a disability, and there's a very important difference between the two words. Don't ever let anyone treat you as if you were different or handicapped."

Later that day, we met a lovely 22-year-old girl who had lost her leg to cancer a few years before. She had been through chemotherapy and was doing well. She did not volunteer what type tumor she had.

She laughed as she tossed her head to show off her long, black, luxuriously curly hair and said, "This is my chemo hair. My natural hair was dishwater blonde and straight."

Her name was Ellen. She had a slight, though distinct limp but was poised and confident in her movements. She walked slowly and gracefully on her prosthetic leg, smiled, and held her head high. Ellen answered many of Ross's questions concerning chemotherapy, and while she withheld no truths about what she had experienced, just looking at her and hearing her story gave Ross hope and confidence.

We returned to our hotel barely ahead of the onslaught of the 5:00 p.m. rush hour.

"Give me your car keys, Mom. I want to go out—alone."

"Wait until we get home. The traffic is awful out there."

"No, I want to go now."

"But you're not familiar with the streets around here. Where would you go?"

"Mother, I am not stupid. Give me your keys. Please."

"You can wait just a few more days until you can practice in the neighborhood at home."

He picked up the keys and walked out.

The following day, Ross returned to Occupational Therapy to be fitted with his first prosthesis. It was a temporary device, all plaster and straps, and he received instructions on how to move his arm to open and close the hook. Straps with metal rings crossed on his back, went under his right arm and over the right shoulder. Nothing about the apparatus could be called pleasing or attractive, but Ross looked better having something instead of nothing where his arm once was.

When we returned to the surgery clinic, Ross was dismissed to go home. The oncologists would call him with the results of the random selection for chemotherapy.

I drove my car to the long-term parking lot of NIH and caught a shuttle back to the hotel. While Ross was out with Mary that evening, one of his friends from Mobile telephoned and said, "I don't know how to ask this, but we've been talking about how Ross looks without his arm. We're wondering, does he have anything at all there?"

I explained to him about the prosthesis but told him I didn't know if Ross would be wearing it. He said there had been conversation and debate among his friends as to the best way to handle their first meeting with Ross.

Around NIH, it's not too shocking to see someone without a limb and, most of the time, we could accept the stares. However, away from the hospital, in a hotel or restaurant, or while strolling in a shopping mall, it was awkward and painful.

By closely watching people's faces, I discovered that they first registered shock when they saw the empty space where the arm belonged. Their eyes shifted to Ross's face, then they quickly looked at me.

When I put a smile on my face—an artificial one—and lifted my chin, most people smiled back and said "hello." At last, I had discovered something I could do for Ross which would be helpful. I could smile. From then on, whenever we walked together, I tried to keep this expression on my face. Because of this phony smile, I gained a reputation I didn't earn. In a place like NIH, troubled souls gravitate toward any appearance of strength and serenity and, without being aware of how it happened, I found myself with many new friends.

4

The next morning in the hotel, I practiced this artificial smile in front of the mirror on the dresser while Ross was in the bathroom, struggling to master the art of getting dressed while using only one hand. But he had not learned how to tie his shoes.

"That's not tight enough, Mom," he said, as I knelt in front of him. "Make the knot real tight so it won't come loose."

"How about a double knot like when you were little?"

"No, Mom. I can't untie a double knot. I've only got one hand, you know."

When I stood, I reached for the button on his shirt.

He jerked away. "I can button my own shirt."

He walked back into the bathroom to tuck his shirt in his pants. He bent down, stretching his left arm, trying to hold his pants up with his elbow. With his right hand, he pulled and jerked the waistband together and finally got it snapped. Part of his shirttail bunched out over the waistband in the back.

"Look at this, Mom. Does it look all right?"

"Let me tuck in this spot..."

"I didn't ask for your help. I asked if it was tucked in."

"Excuse me—I beg your pardon. We're almost out of time."

"Get used to it, Mom. It's going to take me longer to do a lot of things. Remember that, will you please." He tried to reach around his back to smooth the shirt.

We rode the hotel shuttle to NIH, then boarded their van for the ride to the airport. When we reached the terminal at Dulles, Ross took my ticket and checked us in at the counter. He tossed my luggage on the stand, turned around, and handed me my ticket.

"Your boarding pass is already in there. Don't lose it. Put your ticket in your purse," he instructed.

"I think I can take care of my ticket, Ross. What about yours? Do you want me to keep it, too?"

"Mother!" he hissed, as he glared at me. "I've told you a hundred times...."

He strode several feet ahead of me as we moved toward the security gate. When he stepped through, the buzzer sounded and two guards stepped forward.

"Step over here, please," a tall, thickset man called as he waved his scanner at Ross. Ross walked over to him and held up the end of the prosthesis so he could examine the metal hook. One of the guards started scanning across his back.

"There are straps across my back that have metal rings and buckles," Ross said.

The other guard began to hand frisk from his ankles to his neck, then said, "You'll have to take your shirt off."

"You can feel the metal clips," Ross said.

"Remove your shirt."

The crowd of passengers seated in the waiting area made an effort not to watch, turning the pages of their newspapers and magazines with only a quick glance at the scene.

Ross turned his back to the audience and unbuttoned his shirt. The guard lifted the shirt in the back and inspected the harness.

"Lift your arms."

Ross rolled his eyes upward and complied.

When they were satisfied that he wasn't carrying contraband or a deadly weapon, they walked away. Ross re-buttoned the shirt, keeping his head down and his eyes on the floor. He didn't try to tuck the shirt in.

"I'm going to register a complaint with Republic Airlines," I said. "That was absurd."

"No, you're not," Ross whispered. "Forget it."

"There is no reason for all this hullabaloo."

"It's not the airline's fault. It's the airport regulations. Remember, this is an international airport."

"They're taking it too far. Can't they see? You're not trying to hide anything. They're just throwing their weight around—trying to show how important they are."

"They are important, Mom. Do you want to get hijacked to Cuba?"

"There's no reason to go through this. I'm going to complain to somebody."

"Did I ask you to help? I'll let you know if and when I need your help. You'd only make it worse if you make a fuss about it, so drop it, okay?"

As I sat down near the boarding gate with a magazine in front of my face, I rehearsed what I would like to say to airport officials. Ross walked over and sat beside me.

"You want to do something for me? Right now, I need you to tie my shoes again. They're coming loose."

We were unable to sit together on the plane and I took a seat several rows behind Ross. The attendants were hurriedly going through their routines of getting passengers seated and settled in preparation for take-off. When the plane leveled off and food trays were handed out, I experimented with trying to do everything with my right hand only—unwrapping the container, opening the utensils packet, cutting the meat, spreading the mustard. I craned my neck but couldn't see if Ross was eating.

We met in the Atlanta terminal and rushed to our connecting flight, finally sitting together. When we arrived at the Mobile airport, a large group of Ross's friends awaited him and whisked him off to someone's house for a welcome-home party, leaving Bill and me to wait for the luggage.

∾

The next day, Ross decided to go grocery shopping with me. As we walked out to Bill's car, he said, "Let me have the keys. I'm driving."

"No, I'll drive."

"I can drive, Mom. I can handle an automatic transmission. Be real."

"I'm not ready for this—some other time, please. I'm going to the meat market on Airport Boulevard and that's a challenge under any circumstances."

"Give me the keys, Mom. I need to practice. I'm not having you or anybody else driving me around."

As I handed him the keys, I tossed up a quick prayer.

He took the corners faster than necessary, and after he turned into the traffic on Old Shell Road, he let go of the steering wheel while he reached up to adjust the mirror. Then he tuned the radio to his favorite station.

"Why don't you pull over to the curb until you get everything fixed like you want it?" I asked.

"Why? What's your problem?"

He reached for his ever-present plastic cup and sipped a Coke as he turned the curves on McGregor Avenue. On a long stretch of straight street, he reached up, turned the mirror where he could see himself, and began brushing his hair off his forehead.

"That's enough!" I said. "You're being reckless. Either you keep your hand on the wheel or stop and let me drive. You don't have to impress me anymore."

"I am not being reckless! Don't criticize my driving—I'm a good driver. I can control the car just fine, using my left knee. Watch..."

"I don't want to watch and if you don't stop this, I am going to drive. Do you understand?"

"Cool it, Mom! Why are you so uptight? I'm still a better driver than you. You scare me when you drive. You're too slow and poky. You've never learned how to jump into the traffic when you're suppose to."

"I've never had a wreck," I said.

"I've never had one either, don't forget. And, Mom, please remember that I'm trying to learn everything all over again. I've got to learn. You've got to learn to let me. I'm sorry if it upsets you."

～

After we arrived home and unloaded the car, we had visitors from Lucedale, Mississippi. Lana Dungan and her mother Ann had heard of Ross's problem and wanted to share Lana's experience. Lana, 15 years old, had lost her arm to osteosarcoma almost two years before. She had one sister, and their family lived near Ross's aunt Jean and her husband, "Uncle Bud" Persons.

Lana, a cute, vivacious teenager, wore no prosthesis. The tumor had been located in her shoulder, and her entire arm and part of her shoulder had been removed.

When Ross walked into the room, she said, "Hi, I'm Lana. I see we have something in common."

"Yes," Ross said. "It looks that way. When did you lose your arm?"

"December 9, 1980."

"Where did you go? Where did you have surgery?"

"Oschner's in New Orleans. It's a wonderful place—the greatest doctors and nurses in the world."

"Did you have osteo?" Ross asked.

"Yes," she said, shaking her head. "It's an experience, isn't it?"

"You can say that again."

Ann Dungan looked at me and said, "We had never heard of osteosarcoma. You can't imagine the shock when we were told. Well, actually, I guess you can."

"Ross, you'll do fine," Lana said. "I can do almost everything by myself."

"Really? I'm getting used to it. I found out I can drive the car," Ross said.

"I play in the band—march on the field and everything else. You just have to learn a few tricks and adapt as you go along. Are you going to have chemotherapy?"

"I don't know yet. My name is in the pot and if I get selected, I will. Did you have treatment?"

"Yes. I'll tell you about it sometime."

Ann agreed. "There's no point in talking about it until you know if you're going to get it."

Ross and Lana continued to talk about school work, friends' reactions, future hopes and dreams, and, when the Dungans rose to leave, Lana reiterated her love for her doctors. Then she added, "Ross, you've got to have faith. I pray, and lots of people are praying for me."

Early in the following week, Ross received the call from Dr. Poplack, an oncologist at NIH, telling him that the randomization had taken place and he had been selected as one who would not get chemotherapy. Ross had already been pondering the possibility of treatment and decided to visit our friend, Dr. Donald Muller, and get his opinion. He returned three hours later and announced that he wanted to get treatment.

"Why?" I asked.

"Because that's all there is left to do."

"Then call Dr. Poplack back and tell him."

He picked up the phone and reached the doctor immediately, stating his position. Within a couple of hours, Dr. Poplack called again and said there was a 15-year-old boy who lived in Haiti who had been selected for treatment but had refused. The boy and Ross would exchange places in the study. Ross was to be admitted to the hospital five days later.

On Thursday morning as I sat at the kitchen table checking off the long list of things we needed to pack for the return to NIH, the phone rang.

"He was wonderful!" Marilyn said. She worked in the office of UMS Prep School. "It's amazing how he stood before all those people and calmly told his story. You must be so proud of him!"

"I'm sorry...I don't know what you're talking about."

"You weren't there? I can't believe you missed it. Ross spoke to the student body this morning. Didn't you know?"

"No, I didn't. He didn't tell me. He's so shy...I can't believe he would do that."

"Maybe he was nervous, but he certainly didn't show it."

"He should have told me. I would have been there."

He had asked permission to stand in front of the entire student body and tell his story. Marilyn related how he spoke for more than an hour, and how quiet and attentive the students were—even the kindergarten classes. The headmaster canceled the first class of the day.

Ross told of the diagnosis, the tests, and the surgery. He spoke of his fear of returning home with an amputated arm—worried about how his friends might react; afraid they might reject him.

He described NIH—how huge it is—the hundreds of doctors, the laboratories, and patients from all over the world.

He expressed his anxiety about chemotherapy, what he had read and heard. He said he had been told that it could make him very sick, and he would lose his hair. But he had agreed to the treatment because he would be a part of an important study—and it was the only thing left to do.

He ended his speech by telling them that he had given up his arm and was going to take chemotherapy in order to save his life. And he asked for their support.

At a big send-off party at the home of his friend, Jim Phillips, young people spilled out onto the grounds and into the blocked-off street. The Phillips' home, on McDonald Avenue off Government Street in the historic district, rocked with music and teenage chatter. Students from other schools joined UMS class-mates, along with church and neighborhood friends.

Ross left Mobile feeling love he had never experienced before. He had become a symbol—a hero—a role he didn't ask for or want to play.

5

October, 1982

Ross was admitted to the sixth floor of the Clinic Center—the pediatric wing. Osteosarcoma, a pediatric disease, most often occurs in young people between the ages of 10 and 20. Occasionally, we heard of someone near Ross's age or older who developed the condition, but on the sixth floor, if there were any at all, they were not ambulatory.

When we got off the elevator, we entered the hall where Ross would receive chemotherapy. We looked at the scene and felt out of place. Children played on the floor with toys and scooters, and one had learned to do "wheelies" on his IV pole. Parents and nurses darted between them, and Ross and I awkwardly dodged them. A little girl sat at the nurses' station playing with the computer. The "planned chaos" resulted because the children were encouraged to do whatever they felt like doing. Many of them didn't feel like doing anything except remain in their beds because of nausea and vomiting.

Neither the nurses nor the recreational therapists wore uniforms. Energetic, young, and attractive, they were neatly dressed in slacks with sweaters or blouses. Ross responded to them as contemporaries. They were trained in the care of youngsters, and

Ross learned he would receive the same attention which more than compensated for the bother of small children.

His space was a bed in a double room with a 14-year-old boy. A thin plastic-covered pad, a blanket, and a pillow made a bed on the floor for me.

Prehydration with glucose began that night through a needle inserted in a vein in Ross's right arm, which had been strapped to a board, leaving only his fingers free. Looking at him with his only arm immobilized, I knew why my friend in Mobile had said, "You'll have to quit your job." Now, I had a new job description: "primary caregiver"—a yet-to-be defined responsibility.

Chemotherapy had been a vague and obscure word which I had associated primarily with cancer treatment. Ross had investigated during September, and from observation of other patients, it appeared to be a frightful ordeal that took place on the sixth floor of the Clinic Center of NIH in 1982.

The pale, gaunt faces of children, the dark shadows under their eyes, and the absence of hair, eyebrows and eyelashes meant they were in cancer treatment. The only way to guess if they were boys or girls was by the way they were dressed, and even then it was difficult.

Yet, some were laughing and playing, getting into squabbles over a toy like healthy children. A few were downright boisterous, insisting on their way and giving orders to their nurses or mothers. This behavior, often encouraged by the staff, gave the children the feeling that they had a measure of control over their lives, even if in a very small way.

At Ross's request, he was given another conference with the oncologists to ask questions about chemotherapy. He wanted to know what elements were in the drugs, their origins, how they were discovered and manufactured. Finally, the doctors sent a pharmacist to visit him to try to answer his questions.

I attempted to learn how the chemicals act against the cancer and against the human body. Again, my learning was very limited: Because cancer cells are fast growing, drugs are designed to destroy all fast-growing cells. Some fast-growing cells are normal and are found throughout our body, serving many functions which keep us alive and healthy. When these good cells are killed by the drug, the body suffers. Since the drugs do not distinguish between healthy and unhealthy fast-growing cells, they necessarily kill all of them. Some cancer cells are resistant to the known drugs.

With this extremely limited understanding, Ross started chemotherapy, and our knowledge soon increased.

At the beginning of his treatment, we were given a protocol sheet, or a "road map" as they called it, which listed the names of the drugs, the order in which they were to be given, the amounts and strengths of each, and the number of days between treatment.

When I looked at that stack of paper and counted 43 treatments, I didn't fully comprehend, but after estimating the days between treatments, I saw that it would take one year to finish the protocol.

The plan called for seven different chemicals in various combinations and increasing strengths, plus another which served as an antidote—a "rescue" drug—which was to be given for three days following each treatment of one of the drugs. Before each round of chemotherapy, we were asked to sign an "Informed Consent" verifying that we had read and understood all the possible side effects.

The first paragraph stated: "You (your child) are being asked to participate in a clinical study designed to determine the role of chemotherapy in the treatment of this disease and to determine the best timing of chemotherapy."

Further, "Up until the early 1970's, the prognosis for children with osteosarcoma was poor and less than 25% of children survived without developing recurrences of the tumor...Radiation therapy and chemotherapeutic agents (drugs) which are effective in other pediatric tumors are not particularly effective in osteosarcoma...Nevertheless, physicians hoping to improve the prognosis for their patients treated...children with osteosarcoma with the available drugs...there seemed to be some effect in that as many as half of the children treated with chemotherapy after surgery did not develop recurrences. Initially, the improved prognosis for children with osteosarcoma was attributed to the drug therapy which was used. However, more recent studies have cast doubt on this point...As many as 40-50% of children with osteosarcoma diagnosed today and treated with surgery alone may survive without developing recurrence. If this is true, then chemotherapy has contributed very little in the treatment of osteosarcoma. On the other hand, the actual contribution of chemotherapy to improved survival may be substantial. Unfortunately, there are many side effects of chemotherapy which will be outlined below, and some of the drugs will produce permanent side effects.

"Your physician believes there is no way, at the present, to choose whether immediate treatment with chemotherapy after surgery or the delayed administration of chemotherapy for children who develop recurrence is the best treatment.

"There are potential risks and benefits for patients assigned to either treatment group in this study. Patients who receive immediate chemotherapy after surgical removal of the primary tumor, will all be subjected to the real and potential risks of the chemotherapeutic agents...If immediate chemotherapy after surgery is the best form of treatment for this tumor, then the group randomized to receive immediate chemotherapy after surgery will have the benefit of the best treatment.

"Patients randomized to the treatment group receiving no immediate chemotherapy have the potential benefit of avoiding all of the toxic side effects of chemotherapy. Only the children who develop recurrence of their disease, and thus who presumably demonstrate a need for chemotherapy, will be subjected to the side effects of chemotherapy after they have relapsed. On the other hand, patients randomized to the delayed chemotherapy treatment group have the potential risk that recurrent tumor may be more difficult to treat successfully because of the number and size of the recurrent tumors. If chemotherapy does have a beneficial effect in the treatment of osteosarcoma, the chemotherapy may be the most useful before the tumor has recurred and may be less effective for children who have developed recurrences of their tumor...."

Then I began to read about the drugs Ross would be given:

"Chemotherapy. The drugs that will be used for patients who are to receive chemotherapy are listed below, along with possible side effects associated with each. Because these drugs will be given together we anticipate that there will be more side effects....

"1. Methotrexate. This is administered intravenously over four hours. Its side effects include nausea, vomiting, depression in the blood counts, kidney damage, mouth ulcers and diarrhea. The antidote to methotrexate is leucovorin which is administered orally 24 hours after the methotrexate begins....

"2. Adriamycin. This drug is administered intravenously and if it escapes from the vein it may cause burning and destruction of the skin. Anticipated side effects include nausea and vomiting, ulceration in the mouth, diarrhea, blood count depression, loss of hair and liver abnormalities. One important side effect of adriamycin is damage to the heart. In order to minimize the heart damage, the cumulative dose of adriamycin will be limited. It should be noted that if the heart damage occurs, it may not be reversible.

"3. Bleomycin. This drug is administered intravenously. It may cause mouth ulcers and increased pigmentation of the skin.... These side effects are reversible. Bleomycin may also cause lung damage when given in high doses; however, the doses of bleomycin used in this treatment plan are unlikely to cause this complication. Lung damage, however, may be irreversible if it does occur. Fever and chills also accompany the use of bleomycin in some children.

"4. Cyclophosphamide. This drug is administered intravenously. It causes nausea, vomiting and hair loss, as well as depression of the blood counts. Cyclophosphamide may also cause bleeding into the urine....Fibrosis of the bladder may also occur and this effect is not reversible. Cyclophosphamide has been implicated as the cause of sterility, particularly in males. Second malignancies have also occurred in patients treated with cyclophosphamide.

"5. Actinomycin D. This drug is administered intravenously and may cause skin burn if it escapes from the veins into the tissues. It may also cause mouth sores, skin rashes, and depression of the blood count.

"6. Cis platinum. Cis platinum is given intravenously. It

causes severe nausea and may cause kidney damage, which if severe may not be reversible....

"7. Allopurinol. This drug shall be given along with the methotrexate. Its side effects include nausea in a small proportion of patients and skin rashes."

Before the bag of chemicals was added to the IV pole, it was necessary to go through prehydration for several hours, and now, two and one-half weeks after surgery, Ross had finished his first prehydration.

The diagnosis and amputation had split the foundation under our family and dropped us into a deep, black hole. The looming chemotherapy was like being in a dark, mysterious, menacing, and slippery cave. Although we were assured that Ross would be carefully monitored, this was a very hazardous undertaking. Regardless, it was time to start the journey and we would have to grope our way along in the dark, not knowing what to expect.

On that Monday morning, while waiting for the nurse to bring in the drugs to begin the first treatment, we were tense and silent, expecting at any moment to have the procedure started. Ross sat on the side of the bed for awhile, then got up, pushed the IV pole with his foot, and stood at the door, looking right and left along the hall. He maneuvered the pole back and forth to the window and made several trips to the bathroom.

We were startled when a trigonometry teacher walked into the room carrying a stack of books. She looked like a schoolmarm wearing horn-rimmed glasses, her gray hair pulled back in a bun. Ross wasn't paying much attention, but she continued to discuss his plan of study. When Andy Tartler came in, she left.

"How's everything in the sunny south?" Andy asked.

"Okay, I guess," Ross said. "I was pretty busy while I was home."

"How's school? Did you get everything lined up so you can keep up?"

"I don't know. I'm not worrying about it right now."

"I can understand why. Other things on your mind, I imagine."

"Is it definite I'll lose my hair?"

"Nothing's definite, Ross. You're old enough to know that," Andy said.

"Is there anything to prevent it?"

"A lot of things have been tried, like keeping icepacks on your head. Doesn't sound too comfortable to me, though. Try to remember that there are fast-growing cells on your scalp, and when the hair falls, it just means that the drug is doing what it's supposed to do."

"There's nothing I hate worse than being nauseated and throwing up," Ross said. "It's the worst feeling I can think of."

"Who knows, Ross, maybe you won't get sick. There are all kinds of psychological games patients play and some of them have had some degree of success."

"Would it be better to not eat anything so I won't have anything to throw up?"

"There again, it varies. Some say they do better when they have something in their stomach rather than taking it while empty," Andy said. He leaned over and placed his hand on Ross's shoulder. "Can you just stop worrying about it? If you feel like throwing up, have at it! And if you don't, so much the better. Just hang loose and let come what may."

"It would be embarrassing," Ross said.

"In this place? You've got to be kidding! That's the name of the game around here. Relax, nobody will pay any attention whatsoever."

"If I make up my mind that I'm not going to be sick, do you think it will work?" Ross asked.

"Doesn't hurt to try," Andy said.

Seeing Ross's nurse at the door, Andy rose to leave. "See you later. I'll be around if you need me."

The cute, peppy young nurse walked into the room carrying bottles of various colored liquids. Humming a currently popular song, she proceeded to hang the bottles on the IV pole, adjusting clamps on the tubes. "Here we go, Ross," she said. "Welcome to the club!" She tossed her head, swinging a long blonde ponytail, as she moved around the room. "This is your initiation ceremony. Sorry it's not champagne or at least a Coors in these bottles. Buzz me if you need anything or have any questions." She skipped out of the room on her way to the next patient.

I sat in a chair near the head of Ross's bed.

Ross stared up at the ceiling and said, "Mom?"

"What is it, Ross?"

"It feels funny."

"Like how? What do you mean?"

"I can tell there's something going into my body that doesn't belong there."

He closed his eyes and lay still throughout the treatment but he wasn't asleep. By 12:30 p.m., the bottles were empty, and after 1:30 p.m., he roused a bit.

"So far, so good," he said. "Maybe I'll be one of the lucky ones."

At 2:30 p.m., the heaves began and he vomited almost continuously until 7:30 p.m.—five hours of constant retching.

With his right arm taped stiffly to a board, he couldn't lift himself from the pillow or hold the emesis basins which the nurse had thoughtfully stacked high before she left. I called for help and a nurse stayed with us most of the time during his first experience with the drugs referred to as BCD: bleomycin, cyclophosphamide (cytoxan), and actinomycin D.

The next day, while waiting for the second round of BCD, Ross said, "Mom, I don't think I'll be sick this time."

"Good. I sure hope you're right. Do you have a game plan to avoid it?"

"No. That's not it. Yesterday, Andy's aftershave lotion was what started the nausea. I could still smell it after he left."

"Should I mention it to him?"

"No, I don't want to hurt his feelings or make a fuss about it. I liked his aftershave before I got sick. There was a lady doctor in here last night during rounds and her perfume was awful. Please don't you ever wear any perfume. Okay?"

Andy would be grieved if he knew how the fragrance affected Ross. Nurses were careful about this for the most part; however, often some of the doctors were not. Visitors and some staff members were the worst offenders. Maybe there should be a big sign on the hall door in several different languages:

"NO FRAGRANCE ALLOWED BEYOND THIS POINT."

As Ross went further along the protocol, he learned that Noxema medicated cream had a pleasant odor. Ivory bath soap and Johnson's baby powder were also acceptable because of their smell—or perhaps the memories.

The same three drugs were given again with the same dreadful results. These two encounters caused Ross to sink into a dark gloom and despondency. He wanted to go home.

Surprisingly, he got his wish. His doctor told him he could be dismissed from the hospital to a hotel the next day, and when he felt up to traveling, he could go home for a few days.

The National Institutes of Health paid Ross's travel expenses plus a stipend to help defray hotel costs, since he was participating in a study. If Ross had been under the age of 18, or if he had been wheelchair bound or too sick to travel alone, NIH would have also paid for my plane fare. No provision had been made for an attendant for an 18-year-old patient who had his arm amputated, regardless of his immobility during chemotherapy treatment and his sickness for several days afterward. However, his plane fare helped our situation and freed him from debate about the practicality of returning home for a few days.

The unexpected news that he could go home required a fast study of logistics and a flurry of action. We soon learned that in order to survive, we had to be flexible—at any moment, our plans could change drastically. I had packed lots of clothes for sea-sonal changes, and, since we were going to be home for only a few days, I repacked, leaving what I could in the trunk of the car to be left at NIH. School materials were left in the classroom.

We had only one night to remain nearby in a hotel, so I chose the least expensive one I could find, reasonably close by. About 10:00 that night, Ross announced that he was starved. Since he had eaten nothing for three days, I wondered how I had failed to anticipate this. We had nothing in the room to eat and his strong craving was for pizza. We were in a business section of town, right on one of the main thoroughfares, so this would be easy, I thought.

I left him alone and went out, walking around the block to see what might be available. I saw a few cafes along the street with their menus taped to the windows, but none of them listed pizza on its bill of fare. Finally, I came upon the pretty wooden door of a bar which had a menu with pizza at the top of the list.

When I pushed the heavy door open, I faced a flight of stairs going down into a basement. At the bottom of the stair, I entered and asked the bartender if I could order a pizza to take out.

He looked me over and said, "Wait here."

The piano music I had heard when I entered became softer and softer, then stopped abruptly. I stood uncomfortably in the stares of several men whose voices became quieter.

The bartender returned and said, "Yes, you can order a pizza to take out. What do you want on it?"

I gave him my order and thought he would ask me to sit, but he didn't. Nervously, I stood for what seemed like an eternity. Finally, I received the pizza, paid my check, and walked back up the stairs into the street.

A few weeks later, I relayed the story to one of the nurses at NIH. She laughed and informed me that I had stumbled into one of the better known gay bars which happened to be in a very rough neighborhood. I had never heard of a gay bar.

At that time, it was not a laughable matter to me, but I remembered that the pizza was delicious. Ross ate his first food in several days and slept well. The next day, we loaded all our possessions in the car, drove it back to the NIH parking lot, and went by shuttle to the airport.

Bill met us at the Mobile airport, and when we drove into our driveway, Ross got out and sauntered about in the front yard, looking around as if he were in a strange place. He commented on the falling leaves and the smell of the sweet olive shrub near the side door. He picked up the cat, Mitty, and walked into the kitchen, then through the other rooms downstairs. When he walked out on the patio, he released the cat to chase a squirrel. Then he returned to the kitchen and asked, "Where's Scott? Did you say he had moved on the campus?"

"Yes, he did. He'll be by to see you later. Do you want to open this stack of mail?"

He sat at the kitchen table and opened all the envelopes, carefully reading every word of every card. Then he turned to me and said, "I guess everybody's heard about me."

"Does that bother you?" I asked.

"No, but I won't have time to write everyone back. I have a lot to do at school, and I have to find a doctor here in Mobile."

"People don't expect you to write back. And your appointment has already been made with a doctor. Dr. David Clarkson is highly recommended to us by other doctors."

That night, I said to Bill, "You need to go with us to see Dr. Clarkson."

"Why?" he asked. "I really don't have time, you know. I'm behind in my work as it is."

"But you don't know much about this scene, and Ross and I both really need you to know so you can understand."

"I don't know how you expect me to work, pay all the bills, and be involved in all this. Someone has to worry about money— I can't do everything. The expenses are mounting up, you know."

"Isn't there enough from the sale of the beach property and the club membership to carry us for awhile? Ross and I aren't being extravagant."

"The beach property sale hasn't closed yet, and I doubt American Express would be willing to wait. And secondly, there are other big demands besides yours and Ross's expenses."

"As usual, you haven't discussed your business with me. How could I know?"

"I didn't want to worry you."

"But now you tell me. I don't know why you picked this time to bring it up."

"Look, I'm doing the best I can. Just watch your expenses."

"All right, all right. But, regardless, I think the least you could do is meet Dr. Clarkson. You might have to contact him sometime."

Bill drove us to Dr. Clarkson's office—a refurbished row house on a narrow street by Lyons Park. The waiting room was packed with mostly elderly patients. When Ross was called, Bill and I went with him into the private office at the back of the building which I surmised had formerly been a bedroom.

A young man, Dr. Clarkson sat at a desk with his glasses resting on the end of his nose. Somber and unsmiling, he studied Ross's records which we had brought from NIH. He looked at Ross above his spectacles and said, "What are they trying to do, Ross? Kill you before you get started?" Then he curved his swivel chair around and gazed through a window. When he turned again to Ross, he said, "I'll be glad to follow the protocol. However, if anything arises unexpectedly, I will use my own judgement."

"That's what I would want you to do," Ross said.

"Very well," said Dr. Clarkson. "I'll expect to hear from you each time you're home."

The critical phase of chemotherapy treatment is about ten days after the drug is given, when the blood counts drop. Careful monitoring is essential. When Ross drove himself to see Dr. Clarkson again the following week, he learned what the different white and red count numbers should be under normal circumstances, and he tried to understand everything about his blood that he needed to know. An important factor was that when the white blood count dropped, Ross had no ability to fight infections. Caution had to be exercised in cutting fingernails and brushing teeth. A cut or scratch had to be watched carefully. A temperature of over 100 degrees required immediate hospitalization with antibiotics given for five days intravenously.

On his way home from Dr. Clarkson's office, Ross stopped at school for sessions with his teachers. Only two days remained before he had to return to the hospital in Maryland.

6

Always, before admission to the hospital, Ross had to find out if a bed was available. Often, patients wait several hours in the admitting office, but that time, Ross was lucky.

Prehydration started at 4:00 p.m., and at 11:00 p.m., another one of the chemotherapy drugs—methotrexate, also known as "mellow yellow" by the patients and staff—was hung on the IV pole. It took four hours for the huge bottle of amber liquid to empty into his vein, and before it had finished, vomiting began. This drug was followed by the "rescue"—calcium leucovorin—every six hours for several days.

After discharge from the hospital, we checked into a little motel in nearby Rockville. In addition to our luggage, we hauled in all Ross's paraphernalia from the hospital—medications, books, emesis basins, urine collection bottles, thermometers, and a briefcase full of instructions.

Our accommodations at this motel were adequate but not pleasant or comfortable. It was a "suite" with a separate bedroom for Ross and a sofa-bed for me in a room with a semi-kitchen. Whenever he became hungry, I thought I could prepare something for him, any hour of the day or night. After a trip to a grocer and locating some of his favorite foods, I found out the

stove didn't work. But it really didn't matter. The effort was useless because he couldn't eat anyway; yet he was famished.

During the first night there, he got up and walked into the
bathroom, crossing through the room where I had been sleeping.
I thought nothing of it until the next morning when I went into
the bathroom. There, on a towel, he had placed most of his beautiful auburn hair.

It's not important, I told myself. It's only hair.

The looks of his hair had been part of our conversations since
he was old enough to talk. When he was a child, he was teased
about his red hair, and he hated the nickname, "Red." One day, he
climbed into my lap, crying because of the frustration of having
red hair.

"Mom," he said, "if I pray to God, would he change the color
of my hair?"

Ross had many of the personality traits often associated with
red hair, but he didn't use temper tantrums to get his way and he
didn't fight with his friends. I tried to reassure him that God
could do anything.

Neither of us mentioned his hair loss, but the next day, we
went to a mall across the street where he bought a classy tweed
hat, using gift money given to him by a Sunday school class.
Mary managed to get two painter's caps from *The Washington
Post* with lettering across the front exactly like their newspaper
name.

Those days in the cheerless motel were difficult for both of us.
Sometimes Ross verbalized his anger, fear, and frustration. At
other times, he sulked and refused to talk. Physically, he felt
wretched. Often, when thinking out loud, he said, "I've got to do
the best I can."

His dreams of independence from home, parents, and school
authorities had faded. Now, at 18 years old, he was catapulted
into a scary, sick world, hip-to-hip with his hovering mother.

"Do you need anything?" I asked.

"No. I'll let you know if I do."

"Have you taken your temperature?"

"That's my job, Mom. I don't need you to remind me."

"I haven't seen you take it. You have to check it three times a day, remember."

"I heard what they said. I know what to do. I'm not a little kid, you know."

"You feel okay?"

"No, I don't feel okay."

"Sorry. Can I do anything? I'll be glad to go out and get anything you want."

"I'd like you to go out for awhile. But don't stay gone long."

"I don't need anything, Ross. I don't have to go out."

"Please, Mom. I want you to leave. Go get me something. I don't care what you get. Surprise me."

"I'm not a mind reader, Ross. I don't know what would make you feel better."

"Neither do I, Mom. You've got to do the best you can."

I left the room and returned in an hour. "Was I gone too long?"

"Not long enough. Did you bring me anything?"

"I have some magazines and a chocolate milk shake."

"You know I can't drink a milk shake. You can have it. What magazines did you get?"

I handed him the bundle and started back out the door. "I'm going to walk around the neighborhood for awhile."

"How long will you be gone?"

"Not long—just a few minutes. Okay?"

"Don't go very far."

Stay gone a long time, but don't go far.

After being quiet for several hours one day, he said to me, "You know, Mom, I've been thinking. If I had to lose a limb, I'm really lucky it was my left arm. I'd rather lose an arm than a leg— and it could have been my right arm. I still have my elbow which makes the prosthesis more useful. I can move around and go wherever I need to. I'd hate not being able to walk and go where I want to."

Any time Ross had any symptom whatsoever—a cough, runny nose, or an ache or pain, a little alarm went off in my head. Was it caused by chemotherapy—or could it be cancer? It was a real fear based on things I had learned from other caregivers when they spoke of their children's symptoms preceding a relapse.

The recent treatment of methotrexate caused much more havoc than the doctors had anticipated and, according to the protocol sheet, it would be given one day a week for four weeks, increasing the strength of each successive dose.

Any time he felt like eating, we selected a restaurant nearby and got out of the dismal motel. Ross's adventurous nature led us to all the ethnic restaurants in the area. At his favorite Italian cafe, the Bello Mondo, we found tasty and filling dishes which were relatively inexpensive.

After the next round of methotrexate, we rechecked into the same motel loaded down with the same instructions and supplies. The side effects became worse, and new ones appeared. Sores developed in his mouth and throughout his digestive system. We returned to the hospital daily for blood work, throat cultures, and various medicines for each problem.

It rained for days. Both inside and outside of our motel, there was little relief from the buffeting of the distressing and depressing atmosphere.

Sickness and inactivity was a foreign state for Ross. By nature, he had been a take-charge person and a problem solver. From an early age, he showed decisiveness with a streak of stubbornness. Our biggest problems in the past had developed when I questioned his high-flown ideas or tried to slow him down on some plan he had in mind.

He had been enthusiastic and sensitive and had no difficulty expressing love for people. In many ways, he was a visionary, always planning how to improve something. Often, I thought he did things just to prove they could be done.

If maturity can be gauged by the ability to delay gratification, then he could be considered mature. He had short-range plans and long-range goals with the ability to be totally lost in the project at hand, yet never taking his eyes off some future, distant goal.

Although his grades in school were only average, he had a keen intellect and often pored over things unrelated to school work. Before he even began school, paleontology and astronomy occupied his thoughts. From infancy, he required extra effort to respond to his needs and interests.

As a child, he was confidently assertive. Yet, he had many friends and playmates, so I knew this aspect of his personality was reserved primarily for me. I never saw him bully a playmate, but noticed that he usually did the planning and directing of whatever activity was going on. He served as ring leader in both the acceptable and questionable activities and relished his role of "king of the mountain."

His best childhood friend, Alex Lankford, also had red hair and similar temperament. They met in kindergarten and were inseparable for many years. When they disagreed, which happened often, they reminded me of two men debating an issue with point and counter-point, always with kindness and awareness of the other's position. They were often at complete odds with each other, but were courteous and never became angry. They concocted secret plans and, when together, needed a watchful eye.

They both fell in love with their third-grade teacher, and before Christmas, they saved every penny they could find for their shopping. They pooled everything they had and spent their entire savings on a gift for the teacher.

Before they walked down the street to her house, they washed their faces and combed their hair, but when they reached her door, they lost their courage. When she looked out her window and saw them sitting on the front step, she opened the door. After quickly handing her the gift, they ran back home again.

These poignant memories rolled like a film before me as I looked out into the gray, gloomy rain in Maryland.

Often, I felt utterly worthless in this role of primary caregiver. The more Ross tried to tell me what he wanted me to do, and how to do it, the more I failed.

He was too weak, dizzy, and nauseated to drive the car, but still managed to keep his eyes on the traffic while I drove. "Go on, Mom! A yellow light doesn't mean stop. Somebody's going to ram us from behind. You've got to move!"

"Be quiet while I'm driving."

"And you don't have to wait till the streets are completely

clear from here to Baltimore before you move. Jump on in and speed up!"

"Will you shut up? It doesn't help for you to yell at me."

"I am not yelling! Get ready, you've got to change lanes soon. Put your left blinker on; watch your mirrors. Look out! Watch what you're doing! We're going to get hit!"

"If you don't be quiet, you may find yourself on the side of the street with your thumb in the air. Just shut up!"

"Who taught you to drive? And where did you learn? Probably in some hick town filled with little old ladies."

"Yeah, you're right. My dad taught me when I was thirteen years old—on gravel roads in Mississippi—back in the dark ages when we didn't have automatic transmission."

"Well, that certainly explains everything...."

When walking together along the halls of the Clinic Center, the scene was not much different.

"Don't walk in front of me, Mom. You don't know where I have to go."

"Yes, I do, but you go right ahead. Lead the way. I don't care. Take off." I slowed my steps so he could pass me.

"But don't lag so far behind. In this mob, we might get separated. Don't try to walk beside me. The hall's too crowded and you're carrying too much stuff."

As he strode forward, I craned my neck to keep him in sight. "Lead on, my fearless, bossy leader," I whispered.

When he reached the elevator, he turned and looked until he spotted me. "Hurry up," he called. "You're going to make me late."

The elevator door opened and I quickly stepped on, moving to the rear of the car before Ross ordered me to. As soon as we got off on the sixth floor, he turned to me and said, "Didn't you see that patient trying to get on the elevator? You stepped right in front of her."

"There was such a crowd at the door. I'm sorry, I didn't notice...."

"How could you not see someone with a cast on her arm? Will you please pay attention!"

He always had something to give to me to keep for him—an

important record, a book, mail, a slip of paper with a phone number, a fountain pen, or any of the myriad things one collects while around a hospital. Although I had been carrying a briefcase for important papers and schedules of treatment, there were also plane schedules, shuttle schedules, metro schedules, list of motels, map of the city, calendar, stationery and phone numbers, his stack of mail, candy bars, school books and papers. Nevertheless, whenever he wanted something, he expected instant retrieval from this bag of belongings.

In addition to the briefcase, I began carrying a large shopping bag for his medical supplies. Later, I added a plastic hospital bag to carry his prosthesis when he didn't feel like wearing it.

When we left the sixth floor following his next treatment, he couldn't walk because of weakness and dizziness. I pushed his wheelchair along the hall and pulled another one behind us which I had confiscated and loaded with all our luggage and bags of things. We waited a long time for an elevator with enough space for us to get on with our caravan.

Just as there were no orderlies readily available at the hospital to assist if the patient had a caregiver, there were no bellboys at the little motel where we were staying, so the procedure had to be repeated, this time without a wheelchair, and without an elevator. With my arm around his waist, Ross managed to walk into the motel and climb two flight of stairs before collapsing into bed.

After several more trips to the car to unload all our gear, I flopped down in a chair and said, "Whew! That felt like running a marathon. I'm bushed."

"Why do you carry all that junk? You look like a bag lady."

Later, I thought, I can cry. Early on, I learned that it was best if I didn't let him know that I felt tired, sad, worried or angry. Any complaints about anything was interpreted as dissatisfaction. In his position, he saw no reason for me to grumble about anything.

Some of the social workers had witnessed a scene or two between us and they disagreed with my attitude. Andy Tartler stopped me in front of the elevator one day.

"Mrs. Phelps? Could I have a word with you? How's everything?" he asked as he ushered me to a corner.

"I guess everything's okay. I really don't know. Ross is such a bear."

"That's why I want to talk with you. You're not helping Ross by allowing him to take out his frustrations on you. You remember I am Ross's social worker—not yours, so perhaps you might want to talk with Joan about this."

"He's scared, sick—he has a right to be grumpy."

"You're sounding like a martyr. You don't have to pretend you like this. He doesn't need to feel guilty after a tirade."

"I didn't realize he felt guilty. He shouldn't. He's not that way all the time. He's usually very courteous."

"If you allow this to continue, you're going to end up hating Ross and he's going to hate you."

"At times, he does already."

"No, he doesn't. Don't let him take out his feelings on you. As long as he has you, he won't open up to us. He's Mister Nice Guy to everybody else. Everybody loves him."

"He feels safe with me. He knows that, no matter what, I'll keep on loving him. He needs someone to vent his feelings on."

"Right. And that someone is me, not you. When you've had enough, let him know. He won't crumble. He's a strong kid."

The following week's treatment had to be postponed because Ross was too ill to take it. There were conferences and tests, none of which could solidly identify why he was having such a severe reaction so early in the treatment. A week later, the treatment was given and then he had permission to go home again. I juggled plane and shuttle schedules, packed the car to leave at a remote, long-term parking lot at NIH, and got us on the plane.

7

That week at home, Ross couldn't attend school—the ulcers in his mouth had spread to his lips and down his throat. Another problem developed unexpectedly—a heretofore unknown side effect of methotrexate. Large blisters appeared on the bottom of his feet, as if the soles had been scalded in boiling water. Some lesions turned into holes of raw, flaming flesh.

At best, getting dressed and putting on socks with one hand had been awkward and frustrating. It became impossible for him to pull his socks on without scraping across the painful blisters. He spent most of his free week on the sofa, hardly leaving the house unless his friends came to get him. Still, compared to a dismal hotel in Maryland, being home was wonderful.

Thanksgiving came and went without much celebration in our home. The Mothers' Club of UMS provided a traditional Thanksgiving dinner and another friend brought a cake, but Ross was unable to eat anything at all.

Holidays and family traditions were of major importance to Ross. In his kindergarten year, he wanted a Thanksgiving feast, complete with a cornucopia for the centerpiece. He came to the table that year dressed as an Indian.

At his kindergarten's Thanksgiving service, all the little children's classes took turns singing the song they had rehearsed for weeks. Ross's class filed in, nervous and twitching, as they prepared for their moment in the limelight. Ross's voice could be heard above the others as he underscored the words, "We *gather*, *to-gather*, to ask the Lord's blessing..." He was very serious about being thankful *to-gather*.

On this Thanksgiving Day, he resembled pictures of prisoners of World War II. He looked like many other patients on the sixth floor at NIH—and he had only just begun, with still two drugs on the protocol sheet which hadn't even been introduced yet.

                        ∾

December, 1982

Early in the following week, we returned to NIH for the next round of methotrexate, followed the next week by three consecutive days of adriamycin. He went to the out-patient clinic for adriamycin, where he lay on a table as the nurse sat beside him and pushed the drug slowly through the needle. It had few obvious side effects—no nausea—but it had to be limited because of possible irreversible heart damage. It exhausted him, too, and after the third day's dose, he slept in the hotel from early afternoon until the next day.

Checking my calendar, I saw that his next scheduled treatments were December 19th and 26th, which meant Christmas would most likely be spent either in the hospital or in a hotel in Maryland. I called his doctor and got a schedule change so his treatment would be delayed long enough for him to spend Christmas at home. I had our bags packed before I woke him with the good news that he would have two weeks at home.

There were no shuttles to Dulles Airport from NIH on Saturday. The hotel had one, but it was too expensive. Freezing rain, wind, and snow battered Bethesda, so Mary braved the weather and traffic to our hotel where she helped pack, load our car to leave at NIH, then drove us in her car to the airport.

Ross had some experience with air travel before his problem developed, and he enjoyed flying. However, during the previous winter, he, like millions of others, watched intently all the television coverage of the plane that went down in the Potomac River in Washington. After that, he refused to fly in or out of National Airport. Consequently, we had to use Dulles International. The distance from Bethesda to either of the two airports was about equal; however, shuttle service was frequent to National, but not to Dulles. We often relied on Mary to get us to the airport.

When we arrived at home, the family celebrated Scott's 20th birthday on December 13th, the day we traditionally decorated our Christmas tree. Ross lay on the sofa in front of a fire and listened to Christmas music as Bill and Scott brought down the boxes of ornaments and trimmed the tree which they had selected.

Ross managed to go to school for a couple of hours each day the following week before the Christmas holidays began. In the past, he had protested having to wear uniforms; however, he seemed to welcome the opportunity to get back into a regimented, orderly life, even if for a short time. He was permitted to be "out of uniform" so he could wear soft sneakers on his painful feet. They also allowed him to wear a recently purchased dark brown suede hat which became a hallmark for him.

His baldness caused acute distress, but he never discussed it with anyone. His hat became his security—kept close at hand at all times—and often when he was about to leave the house, he'd ask, "How do I look, Mom?"

During assembly one morning, the soccer team called him on stage and presented him with their winning soccer ball, signed by each member of the team and everyone on the opposing team.

During the final week before the holiday, his physical symptoms accumulated and intensified with almost every part of his body suffering in some way.

Mary flew home from Washington on the 22nd and brought Ross two live lobsters in a styrofoam case. Our annual fudge-making tradition took place, everyone in the kitchen with their assigned responsibilities—the mixing, the cooking, beating and sampling. Ross tried to sit at the kitchen table to watch all the activity but soon returned to the sofa in the living room and stared at the flames in the fireplace.

On Christmas Eve, he agreed to give the lobsters to our good friends and neighbors, Hazel and Lewis Mayson, who had offered to cook them. Scott and Mary drove him around town so he could personally deliver a stack of Christmas cards he had made.

When they arrived home, we had our usual seafood dinner, with relatives and friends dropping in and sampling tastes on paper plates. Ross didn't try to taste anything, but his spirits were high for the holiday he loved.

On Christmas morning, we skipped breakfast and planned instead an early dinner. Ross tried to eat lobster but couldn't. He had dreams about food, and he talked of lavish gourmet meals, but even water caused pain in his mouth, throat and stomach.

We had several groups of visitors, including the Riordas from New Orleans. Ross's Aunt Dorothy Riorda—my sister,—her husband Joe, and their children had always visited during the Christmas holidays. The children, Allan, Kathleen, and Susan, and our three children had spent many Christmas holidays together.

A friend of Ross called an impromptu Christmas Day party for him, and his New Orleans cousins drove him there, while Dorothy helped me to clean the kitchen, wash clothes, and pack.

Bill went with us the next day when Ross had to return to NIH for another round of methotrexate. Since it was the holiday season, we upgraded our accommodations to the Bethesda Marriott Hotel.

8

The Bethesda Marriott was quite a contrast from where we had been staying. The spacious lobby was decorated with lighted trees and garlands. We had a choice of three different restaurants. There were indoor and outdoor heated pools and a health club in the basement. Uniformed bellboys and a concierge were close at hand, and an efficient staff smoothed our way.

We were given a spacious handicapped room on the first floor which overlooked the terrace and grounds. Two double beds, a large dresser, stuffed chairs, and a writing table furnished the room, which was decorated in soft pastels of coral and aqua.

By New Year's Day, we had been in Bethesda for four days and Ross's series of treatments made his joints swell and his lips bleed; the ulcers in his mouth and stomach burned torturously. He told the doctors he couldn't take it any more. He was quitting the program.

While standing at the door listening to the discussion, I said, "He had a miserable time while we were home. He's lost so much weight. I don't know how he can continue."

"We would like for him to try a little longer with an adjusted protocol," a doctor said. "Actually, he's done well. The symptoms and side effects come with the territory of this protocol of chemotherapy. He's had no fever to speak of and his lab work is right on schedule—just what we expect."

After the doctors agreed that they would scale the strengths of the drugs back to a more tolerable level, Ross reluctantly agreed to continue.

When Bill left to return home, I set up a makeshift kitchen in the hotel room. I kept a cooler box filled with canned drinks, juices, and milk. I found that by placing a can of soup in very hot water in the lavatory for several minutes, it would be heated to about the only temperature Ross could tolerate.

In spite of the holiday atmosphere of the hotel, Ross remained despondent. I thought of the brochures I had seen in every waiting room at the Clinic Center which stated that efforts should be made by the caregiver to be cheerful when the patient is depressed. I wondered who wrote that. Most of the time, Ross had maintained an extraordinarily optimistic attitude, but now his confidence and determination had slipped. He lay in the bed for hours with his arm across his eyes.

"Mom, I can't take much more of this...I've had it!"

I sat on the side of his bed and placed my hand on his shoulder. "It's up to you, Ross. I understand."

"You don't know what it's like to be sick all the time."

"No, I don't. But I can't tell you what to do."

He sat up in bed and I placed two pillows behind his back. He turned and looked at me with reddened eyes. "Do you think they'd take me back if I drop out?"

"I don't know. We could ask them."

"What if I drop out and then have a metastasis?"

"I can't believe they wouldn't take you back. We can ask."

"But if I drop out, I won't be a part of the study. If I'm not in a study, I can't even be a patient here."

"I can't believe they would turn their backs on you. If you want to drop out, then do it. It won't be the first time or the last time that a patient drops out. The doctors aren't going to criticize you. And what if they do? Who cares?"

"I trust them, Mom, but they're not like regular doctors. You have to follow their protocol. But I can't take it anymore, Mom. I don't know what to do...."

"Remember, we're going to take it one day at a time. Don't assume you're going to feel this bad from now on. This may be the very worst part and you may not feel this bad again."

He suddenly turned his back to me and pounded his fist on the pillow. "Like you said, Mom, you know nothing about it. You don't know how it feels—you couldn't possibly understand, so you might as well not try. Forget I said anything about it."

"I'm trying, Ross. Give me credit for trying."

"Forget it, just forget it. You don't understand. Just go out somewhere. I need to think. Go for a drive or a walk, go shopping, do something, will you?"

"Okay. How long do you want me to be gone?"

"I don't care. Stay as long as you want."

"Need anything before I leave?"

"No."

"Can I get you anything while I'm out?"

"No! Just leave!"

We were together in this hotel room for two weeks before he slowly began to get better. He occasionally labored to get dressed and drove himself around Bethesda.

When he wanted to be alone, I left him, taking long walks in the neighborhood. The hotel was near a residential area with narrow, curving, tree-lined streets. The gently rolling hills caught icy breezes that scattered the leaves. These walks were more than a breath of fresh air. They were moments of freedom and a reminder that there was more to life than being trapped in a hotel room with a weary, angry, sick son. Even if I could have booked an adjoining room, it wouldn't have made any difference. Both of us were exhausted—physically, mentally, and emotionally. He was tired of me, and I of him, and we were both consumed with fear and worry. We needed to be far, far away from each other.

Often, when I returned from my walk, he would ask why I stayed gone so long. Once I drove to get milk shakes and, when I left the restaurant, I couldn't get the car to start for 30 minutes. When I finally got back to the hotel, he seemed to be in a panic and was very upset with me. Eventually, I figured out that he wanted me out of the room but close by so I could check often to see if he needed me. I moved my crossword puzzles to the lobby.

One night, unusually tired, I dressed for bed early, curled up in a chair, and scanned a *Reader's Digest*—short stories which held my attention long enough to finish.

Ross sat in bed—prosthesis off, barefoot, dressed in gym shorts and tee shirt—as he watched television.

"Mom, would you go to the drink machine and see if they have a root beer?"

"No, I'm not going through the lobby in my robe."

"Come on, Mom. It's not like I'm asking a big favor. Big deal. Can't you do anything I ask?"

"Go get it yourself."

"I'd have to get completely dressed—put on my prosthesis, shoes, everything."

"I'm not walking through the lobby. There are parties going on all over the hotel. People are all dressed up. Forget it."

"You sure do care a lot about what people think."

"So? Forget it. I'm not going. There's something in the cooler box if you're thirsty."

"I'm sick of Cokes. They make my stomach hurt. You sure are grouchy tonight."

"I am not. I'm tired. You're being unreasonable."

"Unreasonable? Just because I asked you to get me a root beer? Gee, I'm so sorry if I'm such a bother to you."

"That's enough, Ross. I don't want to listen to this."

"Then listen to yourself, Mom. You should listen to what you're saying. I thought you wanted to be here to help me. But no, you can't do me one little favor."

"Ross, please just shut up!"

He slapped the button on the TV set, turning it off. Snatching his socks off the bed, he pulled them over his feet, wrong side out. He reached into the closet, grabbed a shirt, rattling the hangers. When he put his arms through the straps of the prosthesis, he pulled the shirt on, leaving it unbuttoned.

"Come over here and let me tie your shoes."

"No, thanks. I don't want you to do me any favors."

"That's enough, Ross. Shut up!"

"You keep quiet, too," he said before he slammed the door.

He stayed gone a long time. I don't know where he went, but that night I didn't care.

But things blew over, and finally, toward the end of the second week, he could eat real food. We went out to dinner in a nearby restaurant. As we entered, I saw white tablecloths and flickering candles.

"We may be in the wrong place, Ross. This looks expensive."

"Let's check it out. I'm hungry and I think I could eat most anything. I'm ready for a decent meal."

After we were led to a table by the host, Ross stood behind my chair, assisting me before he took his seat.

"This is nice," he said.

"Yes—feels like we're 'dining' instead of eating."

The room was crowded with well-dressed patrons, their conversations muted by upholstered chairs and thick carpeting.

"Can I order a lobster cocktail?"

"Only if you're sure you can actually eat it. Be careful what you order. I'd hate to leave an expensive meal."

Music came from the room next door—a piano playing a medley of my favorites—movie themes, Simon and Garfunkel, show tunes.

He savored the lobster cocktail, rolling his eyes upward in a gesture of relief and delight. The salad followed promptly and he didn't question a single thing that was in it. I spread butter on crackers and placed them on his bread plate.

When his entree came, he said, "Could you put some butter on my potato? I like lots."

"Do you want to hand me your plate and I'll cut your steak while I'm at it."

"I think I can cut it with my fork—it looks tender and juicy. Just fix my potato and bread."

After I handed his plate back to him, he said, "Thanks. This is great. It's the best meal I've had in a long time."

"It's the only meal you've had in weeks."

He caught me with my head turned toward the room from which the music came, nodding to the rhythm.

"Would you like to dance?" he asked.

"What? Me? Dance?...I'd love to."

Ross's dancing experience, mainly at high school functions, was limited. I had never danced with him except for the required "duty"dance after the call-outs.

We approached the dance floor and before stepping on, he said, "I don't know how we're going to do this. Why don't you hold my right hand and I'll see if that works."

Now I understood. He needed me for practice.

We tried his idea but it felt totally backward and we laughed at the awkwardness. I suggested that I place my right hand under his left elbow. I knew he was worried about girls' reaction to the prosthesis, and his arm wasn't strong enough to hold the prosthesis up for long. Resting his elbow in my right hand seemed fine with me, but didn't satisfy him. We tried a few other ideas, none of which pleased him.

We had the floor almost to ourselves with only one other couple moving slowly to the music. The gentlemen danced his partner near to us and smiled while warning us that he might step on our toes. With a few graceful turns on the floor, he moved to the side where he sat his lady in a wheelchair and fastened straps around her useless legs.

When we returned to our table, Ross asked, "Could we come back here again? This is a great place."

"We'll see. Maybe."

He ate a slice of French silk chocolate pie while I sipped my coffee.

"Think you could make a pie like this?"

"Not likely. I'm not all that talented with desserts."

"You make good cakes."

"Thanks. I'm glad to hear I can do something right."

"Mom, let's don't start fussing and fighting again."

"I'm not starting anything—just stating a fact. Nothing I've done lately pleases you."

"I haven't felt very well, you know."

"I know. But that's no excuse to be so cross with me."

"Okay, I'm sorry I've been grouchy. I didn't mean to talk bad to you and hurt your feelings. It's a nice evening. Let's don't spoil it."

"I agree. I'm sorry I lose patience with you. I know you don't feel well and don't like being stuck with me all the time. I understand."

"We've got to do the best we can, Mom. Why don't you talk to your social worker sometimes?"

"Maybe I will. What about you? Do you talk to yours?"

"Sometimes. Most of the time, I don't feel like talking to anybody."

"Neither do I, Ross. But I will go to the group meetings."

When walking the crowded halls of the Clinic Center, overpowering loneliness often assailed me, and I would catch myself searching for a familiar face among the hundreds of strangers. Although I had an assigned social worker, I failed to take advantage of her expertise. The social workers conducted weekly meetings of the caregivers in order to find out if we needed anything or if there were problems or suggestions. In actuality, they hoped the meetings would turn into group therapy. This noble and worthwhile effort rarely paid off because most of the caregivers were so emotionally, mentally, and physically exhausted they didn't have the presence of mind to think about anything except their patients.

From the group, I soon learned that Ross was one of the healthier ones on the hall. One mother related through her tears how her child used her as the target for all the anger, fear, and frustration he felt. I had thought that I was the only one experiencing this devastating result of what I had come to believe were heroic efforts on my part. "Doing the best I could" was not enough.

Obviously, I had achieved a small measure of success in keeping the superficial smile on my face. I became suspect to the staff of social workers. They often checked on me. Once I was invited into a private office to discuss Ross's situation.

She began, "We're here to help in any way possible, and we want you to know we're available. If you don't feel free to discuss your feelings with us or with any of the other parents, I'll be happy to call in some of the parents of former patients and I'm sure you can find someone you can relate to."

I told her I appreciated her interest, but didn't say that I preferred to be left alone. "Who are these parents of former patients? Where do they live?" I asked.

"Actually, they're from all over the country, but we have some who live nearby and we keep in touch with them," she said.

"And their children—how are they doing? What do you mean by 'former patients?' Are they in remission?" I asked.

"Well, no," she said slowly. "The ones I have in mind for you had the same disease as Ross, but they failed to respond to the treatment."

"No. No, thank you. Find someone who has a child with osteosarcoma who is living and doing well. I would love to meet one of them."

She had studied the currently accepted theory of the stages of grief and had me pegged as being in denial. It must have been their theory that if caregivers would acknowledge that their patient was going to die, they would be better able to cope, and that anyone who hadn't accepted their version of that truth was out of touch with reality.

"You simply must face the fact that Ross may die," she said emphatically.

"Not today, I don't," I said, as I left her office.

Another time, I received a distinct message from a social worker, although she didn't verbalize it, that I should "let Ross go"—give him permission to let go of his will to live. I wondered if she thought Ross's recovery possibilities would be strengthened if he knew that it was okay with me for him to die.

I never asked her what she meant. Ross never appeared to me to be ready to turn toward death although it was in the shadows around his mind. But the social worker's words prompted a deep reflection and a little guilt. I wondered if my attitude was causing Ross more pain.

By this era of my life, I had developed the belief that negativity was the opposite of faith, doubt could lead to despair, and that neither negativity nor doubt was a part of love. I believed that those types of attitudes, words, or actions on the part of anyone closely associated with Ross would be detrimental to him. I strove to guard my own thoughts and became irritated with anyone else who expressed a pessimistic outlook. Other people, especially the social workers, mistakenly interpreted my attitude as Pollyanna, assuming that I couldn't face reality. My attitude didn't fit their reality which was based primarily on statistical evidence gleaned from measurable laboratory studies and scientific comparisons. But maybe there could be other factors involved, ones which weren't so clearly and easily measurable. If wanting to hang on to that slender thread of a possibility labeled me as one who avoided reality, then so be it.

If I had truly believed as they did, I couldn't have hidden my thoughts from Ross. I would abhor having someone around me all the time who thought I was going to die—always turning their eyes away to hide their grief and pain. Ross often scrutinized my face, and he saw the grief, pain, and fear. However, I believed the very least I could try to do for him would be to carry the *live* message in my mind, regardless of the statistical evidence to the contrary.

Death, or the likelihood of it, stalked the halls as a constant companion for the staff. The nurses were intimately involved with it. They had an overload of responsibilities and always rushed from one patient to another. In spite of this, they had the courage to smile. They were bright, cheerful, warm, and loving. Their education and training made them experts in giving chemotherapy and attending to the patients' needs.

Often, when on their few minutes break, they used their time to come into Ross's room, pull up a chair, and visit with him, discussing whatever might come to his mind. They touched him, held his hand, or hugged him when he needed it.

I would have gladly done anything to assist a nurse in order to allow her to be free to talk to Ross. Often, I wished for manual labor—anything at all to be useful. We were expected to help. Bathing, bed-changing, food trays, urinals, and emesis basins were our responsibility. Our participation relieved the nurses and made us feel as if we were contributing.

Some mothers, even those with small children, walked out at night and said they couldn't do this 24 hours a day. I could understand. Ross had never had to stay in the hospital for more than two or three days at a time. Some patients had been there for weeks and even months.

A school of thought began to develop that the person emotionally closest to the patient shouldn't be the caregiver. The patient should be protected from knowing that the person he or she loved had to go through this also. The good times were to be shared, not the bad.

This would have been ideal if another caregiver had been available. In most families, no one else was attainable short of hiring round-the-clock private-duty nurses, which few could afford. Often, a single parent with other younger children at home fulfilled this role. Sometimes, the single parent, male or female, also had a job, and could visit their patient only briefly in the evenings if they lived in the area. If they lived a long way away, in many cases, they had to resign their jobs and depend on charity.

The responsibilities of the social workers, recreational therapists, and nurses often overlapped in their efforts to be supportive and helpful to the patients and caregivers. Some of the young people on the staff were there fulfilling internships in several areas of endeavor. Some were in training for psychological and social work. Field work was also done by chaplains of various religious denominations.

The Clinical Associates—the physicians who had responsibility for their assigned patients—rotated, with a new group coming in about every six months. Ross always had two physicians—one in the clinic when he was an out-patient, and one on the hall when he was in the hospital. Invariably, he was assigned to female doctors who were responsible for seeing that he followed the protocol exactly as planned, if at all possible.

Over this group, there were others who committed to a longer period of service, as much as two years. The next level of hierarchy—the permanent staff—planned and followed the study. The chief oncologists made up the top tier of the group. Once each week, the entire group made rounds together and visited every patient on the hall, and also discussed other cases which were not in treatment that week.

The majority of the Clinical Associates were American from all over the United States, but a few were from foreign countries which sometimes caused distress among the caregivers. Learning everything we needed to know about this strange world we were in could be even more complicated by a language barrier. Although the foreign doctors could speak English, often they were hesitant or they used words unfamiliar to the patient. Cultural differences and temperaments also created minor problems.

A young, peppery Italian woman walked swiftly down the halls, her high-heeled shoes clicking on the floor. Once I heard her say in a firm voice, "Don't forget, I am *ze* doctor, you are only *ze* mother, and he must do what I *zay*, not what you *zay!*"

A slender, soft-spoken Oriental girl bowed before approaching the bed. She moved quietly, quickly, and efficiently, then bowed low before leaving the room. She appeared to be so young it was hard to imagine her having graduated from medical school.

India seemed to produce many physicians who studied at NIH; their manner of dress was prevalent in the halls. Mary and Scott had teased Ross about the lovely olive-skinned woman who wore a silk sari in peacock colors. They were also intrigued by the diamond on the side of her nose. On the grounds outside, many men wearing turbans and full length robes walked to and from the cafeteria.

The Associates had a small room near the nurses' station where they caught naps when they could. Every hour of the day or night, a doctor was on the hall. Some of them maintained an aloofness and others were warm and friendly. It wasn't unusual to see a doctor sitting on the floor playing with a child, or picking one up and patting its back in a loving way. I watched a small boy being carried in the doctor's arms because the little fellow didn't want to go for a scheduled appointment.

In the out-patient clinic, an entirely different set of Associates were also on rotation basis. Each day since we returned to Bethesda three weeks before, Ross had been seen in the clinic.

But it was time to start in-patient treatment again, so after hanging around the hospital all day waiting for a bed to become available, procedures were begun to start prehydration.

Because of the assault of the drugs on Ross's body, it had become very difficult for the nurse to find a vein anywhere in his body which was suitable to accept and hold the needle. This became an added problem for Ross since he had to be stuck so often for blood samples, and he became belligerent when the first attempt was unsuccessful. The harder the nurse tried, the more she failed, and often someone from surgery would have to be called in to assist in finding a suitable vein. Once, they gave up on his right arm and found a vein in his ankle.

Ross had to stay in the hospital several days following this treatment, since he had suffered so terribly on the last admission. Again, even though the dosage had been reduced, his joints became inflamed and swollen again. His feet and mouth sores had never gone away. All the doctors had the opportunity to see first hand.

Upon release, we again checked into the Marriott Hotel just before a beautiful, heavy snow. This was a novelty for us, and Ross watched longingly as the huge flakes settled over the pool and terrace. After two days in our warm, pleasant cocoon, the schedule called for another two days of BCD.

Again, Ross wanted to question the doctors about his treatment and asked for a conference in his room. He asked me to leave because he wanted to speak to them privately. I became nervous that he had withheld telling me of some new symptom.

After waiting in the family room for about 30 minutes, I returned. While outside the door, I heard one of the doctors say, "Ross, you do understand, don't you? We're talking about sterility—not impotence. There are thousands of children in the world who are waiting to be adopted...."

As I hurried along the hall, I felt guilty for eavesdropping. But I was joyfully relieved to know that Ross was concerned about living—not dying.

The two days of BCD turned into a nightmare. Everything went wrong. No vein could be found. When the experts came and put the needle in place surgically, it came loose and had to be restarted during the night. Ross had an extreme reaction with hard chills, jerky movements, and sudden, high fever which required immediate IV antibiotics.

When he was discharged to the hotel, I looked at the calendar and saw we had been in Bethesda for one month; January was almost gone. After a couple of nights in the hotel, he dragged himself from the bed and said, "Let's go home."

I jumped on the merry-go-round of packing and logistics and we made our flight from Dulles to Mobile. Again, his friends awaited him at the airport.

9

Ross had never thought himself to be socially popular, but now, caring young people surrounded him. The romances he had been involved in—though ardent and entrancing—were primarily summer beach affairs and a few dates in high school. Now he relished all the attention and affection from the attractive girls who called or stopped by daily.

He attended school that week and spent the rest of his time at home with his visitors. When he walked in one afternoon, pale, tired, and weak, he admitted that he saw no way he could graduate. He was so far behind, and didn't feel up to even trying to catch up. He was also missing all the senior privileges he had looked forward to for so many years.

In addition to all his other problems, his blood count had reached a new low. By the end of the week, his temperature started to rise, which put me into action with my handy thermometer. After his fever went to 101 degrees, he was immediately admitted to the Mobile Infirmary where antibiotics were given intravenously for five days until his fever dropped and the white count started to rise. Having to spend his free week in the hospital in Mobile was the last straw.

Mardi Gras festivities and parades had taken over Mobile as

the faithful had their last fling before the beginning of Lent. Ross didn't want to go back to Bethesda. He called his doctor at NIH and asked that his treatment be postponed one week.

She said, "Absolutely not!"

When he hung up the phone, he said, "Mom, I don't want to go back yet. What's the big deal? I've had to postpone treatment for a week before. She acts like I've asked for a month off. She always gives me a hard time...." He bit his bottom lip and his chin quivered.

"I know, Ross. She acts like some Very Important Person. I call her 'Her Royal Highness.' I guess we're suppose to bow and scrape before Her Honor. Why don't you call Andy and ask him to talk to her?"

He called him and, whether Andy did or not, I don't know, but Ross knew he had an ally. He called The Honorable Doctor back and said flatly that he wouldn't return until the following week. Before he hung up the phone, I heard him say in a loud, firm voice, "You go right ahead. Put me down as an 'uncooperative patient.' I don't care what you put on my record."

No doubt, she had Ross's best interests in mind. But I suspected also that she, like many other doctors involved in his treatment, had an ego that needed to be fed by supervisors. A designation of "uncooperative patient" probably got her off the hook. They were totally focused on the disease and chemotherapy. They had immersed themselves in learning the most minute parts of the body. I often wondered if they ever stopped, stood back, and looked at the person who had the disease.

Ross's friends took him to Mardi Gras parties and parades day and night. He came home only to rest for a few hours, change clothes, eat what he could, then go again. Since we had rigged a scarf for his bald head, fashioned as an Arab headdress, he was in keeping with the many and varied costumes on the streets.

When he came in from the outing on Sunday, he said, "Mom, I need something else to put on my head besides this Arab thing."

"Why? It looks like Mardi Gras to me."

"You're not keeping up with the news in the Middle East, Mom. Trying to look like an Arab isn't in right now."

"Put a cap on top of it. You can be a member of the French

Foreign Legion. How did you manage to stay downtown all day?"

"A lot of my friends' parents have hotel rooms. I went in and rested a lot. We were mostly in Bienville Square."

Bienville Square was the culminating point of the Joe Cain Day Parade and the festivities that followed. Historians established that Joe Cain founded Mardi Gras and organized the first parade in downtown Mobile over 100 years ago. Now Joe Cain was honored yearly with a wild and raucous street party which took over downtown Mobile.

The organized parades and fancy dress balls had been going on almost nightly for weeks. The final three days meant continuous partying in hotels, offices, and in the streets. Jazz and dixieland bands played on street corners, policemen rode horses, curly strings of serpentine tossed from office building windows floated down on the crowd. When the parades passed, thousands of pounds of candy, beads, doubloons, and trinkets sailed through the air as members of various Krewes riding huge, colorful floats rained goodies to the screaming mass of people. Little children sat on their dads' shoulders for a better view as older ones and adults scampered for the beads, baubles, knickknacks and bubble gum. High school bands' music echoed off the tall buildings.

Ross had fun those few days, but more importantly, he learned something: He had choices he could make. He took control. From then on, even though the assault on his body never let up, he made peace with what he had to do and could carry on.

10

Since September, Ross and I had made six trips to Bethesda. Now, in February, 1983, only five months into this cancer-treatment world, it was time for the seventh trip. I had reached the point where I had to admit that both physically and emotionally, I couldn't handle this trip alone, so Bill agreed to go with us. He spent the night with Ross at the hospital following the treatment of methotrexate. But he left the next day, still not knowing what it was like when Ross got the drugs, BCD.

Always, when released from the hospital, Ross never wanted to go straight to the hotel. He had to be outdoors, even if in a car. We drove around Washington and surrounding areas, usually ending up in Rock Creek Park, where he got out of the car and sat on a rock by a rushing, narrow stream. He wanted to breathe fresh air after the unpleasant odors of the sixth floor of NIH.

Another exciting drive was along "Embassy Row," where he watched for limousines, hoping to get a glimpse of some famous foreign dignitary. Occasionally, there were protestors in front of the embassies, with television coverage.

He knew Capitol Hill well and had more driving experience in the District than I, so when he felt like it, he drove me all over the city.

His previous experience in Washington came about the summer before his 16th birthday. He accompanied me there to take care of Mary when she had to undergo extensive surgery on a broken ankle at Sibley Hospital. The idea of leaving a teenage boy at home alone during the day with nothing constructive to occupy him prompted me to take him with me to Washington. Scott had a summer job digging ditches for a plumber, and since he was always a very conscientious worker in whatever job he had, I knew where he would be at bedtime. I didn't have to worry about his evening hours.

Ross had a driver's learning permit, so when we got Mary out of the hospital, he insisted on doing all the driving of Mary's car. Soon after getting her settled in the big Georgetown house which she shared with several housemates, I saw that I wasn't needed. I returned home and left him to take care of Mary.

He helped her at home by doing the laundry, cooking and grocery shopping. He drove her to her office in the early morning madhouse of traffic, made friends with a traffic policeman who let him park the car where he could get Mary in a wheelchair, put the car in her parking space, then wheeled her to her office. Once they reached her desk, he did all her "leg" work. At the end of the day, he got her home and went through the routine again.

When we had left Mobile, he carried his old standby navy blue blazer, so he had to buy a couple of new shirts and ties. He felt very important to be spending his time in a senator's office. He loved every minute of his experience and quickly developed what is known on Capitol Hill as an intern's version of "Potomac Fever." For an almost 16-year-old, Washington was the place to be and he wanted to stay. In spite of his young age, he participated in evening activities with college interns. Once he got Mary settled at home for the evening, he attended receptions and spontaneous parties which abound around Capitol Hill.

Now that we were again in the area, he quickly learned the streets and highways better than I. Once, on a cold, rainy, dreary Sunday, we were out for a drive and he decided he wanted to go to Annapolis.

I gazed at the healthy young cadets near Ross's age as we drove around the campus of the Naval Academy. We walked out on piers to look at sailboats, and had lunch in a seafood cafe on the waterfront. We agreed that the Chesapeake Bay oysters were not nearly as good as the Gulf's harvest.

The next day, we had still another scare when he complained of irregular heart beats and a feeling of pressure in his chest. A rushed trip back to the hospital and examination by a cardiologist revealed nothing out of the ordinary, but from then on, a heart monitor had to be used when he received adriamycin.

That night, Mary and Ross attended a "Mash Bash" in the Stirrup Lounge of the Marriott hotel to watch the broadcast of the final episode of Ross's favorite television show, *M.A.S.H.* There was a costume contest and Ross decided to be a "wounded soldier." For him, this required no costume and aptly described how he looked. However, his battle was a long way from being over.

March, 1983

The following week, he got his permanent prosthesis with the new style, heavy-duty hook. As hard as the physical and occupational therapists worked with him, his upper left arm muscle shrunk very quickly with no hope of ever building it up again or maintaining it in normal size.

"How do like my new hand, Mom?" he asked, moving the prosthesis forward and backward, opening and closing the hook.

"Looks rugged and 'outdoorsy.' What can you do with it?"

"Lots of things. It's strong. I can lift more things than I could with the other one. The other one would bend too easily, but this one won't."

"How much weight will it take?"

"As much as my arm can stand. When I lock it in place, it holds real good. I'll be able to do much more than I could before. I can even tie my shoes with it when I get it in the right position."

"That big thing can clamp on a little shoestring?"

"Yes. Watch," he said, as he bent down, untied his shoes, and retied them. "I've got to practice with it. Maybe it'll help build up my arm. I think I can carry my own luggage with it."

"That's great, Ross. Now you don't need me anymore. Aren't you glad?"

"You can stick around until I get used to it and find out what all I can do. But you don't have to tie my shoes anymore."

Always, on admission, Ross first checked to see if he had any mail. Usually a stack of cards, letters, and packages awaited. He read every message, relishing it as if it were manna from heaven. Knowing of a normal world out there waiting for him, and experiencing the love expressed in the messages, kept his spirits up and his hopes alive.

By this time, Ross knew some of the other patients very well. They, like Ross, were often admitted for a couple of days and then released. Since no one seemed to be following the same protocol in the same time frame, we never knew who would be on the hall at the time of admission.

After handing over his mail to me to add to his collection, he wandered around the hall to see who he could find. Often, it was a sad trip.

For awhile, it seemed that death occurred on the hall about once each week. These tragedies tore into the hearts of the other patients and their caregivers as well as the nurses and staff. There was no way to avoid watching as a broken family gathered their things and walked along the hall alone. We also shared the daily hopes and dreams, and rejoiced at good reports for a difficult case.

Little Jody, a five-year-old with big brown eyes, had put up a long fight in his struggle against leukemia. At the end, his mother stumbled out of the darkened room, supported on each side by nurses. She had kept the vigil for 48 hours.

A young man I had never seen outside his room died from a complication of the treatment while the disease was under control. His weeping mother paced back and forth in the hall as the boy received his final transfusion of blood platelets.

Meg, a 30-year-old mother of three, contracted a pediatric form of cancer. The curtain was always pulled around her bed for the short time she was there. Her husband brought their children to see her the day before she died.

Fifteen-year-old Wendy failed to recover from her relapse of osteosarcoma after having been in remission for almost two years. She never felt like trying to use her prosthesis or bother with a wig. Her leg had been amputated high—near her hip—and she spent most of her time in a wheelchair, gamely going to the teen meetings and pizza parties on the hall.

Sandi, tall and willowy, was a cheerleader, and her mother believed her acrobatics hastened the onset of Ewing's sarcoma. Sandi wore a long blonde wig which matched her real hair. She often wore her team's colors and relished her cheering section back home.

Matt, a football player, also had Ewing's. He, too, wore his team's colors and was full of bravado and confidence that he would win this big one. When he first arrived, he was strong and muscular. He moved about with authority. As the weeks went by, he became pale, thin, and weakened. He and Sandi often walked together, hand-in-hand. Sandi and Matt died a few weeks apart.

Little Robbie died in his home town hospital after spending weeks on the hall. Laura and Paul also chose not to come back when their disease became resistant to treatment.

John Talbert, a young teenager, had Ewing's sarcoma. It was discovered in a rib. Much of his time was in the laminar-flow room, the only necessarily private room on the hall. The plastic barriers to his room required the doctors and attendants to dress in space-age gear. John's mother, Elise, sat outside the plastic window all day every day as well as many nights. Although she always had a smile on her face, her sad, tired eyes betrayed her. John survived his ordeal.

Elizabeth Miller had battled leukemia for several years and had been in remission for a long time when she had a relapse during her freshman year in college. She looked so very frail and ill, and yet she managed to again go into remission. Elizabeth and Ross were near the same age and they both formerly had red hair and the personality that often went with it.

When Buddy Green first visited NIH, I happened to be in the downstairs lobby, where his anxious parents were waiting for him to return from one of his tests. When his diagnosis was confirmed, a small measure of relief and hope came with it. Buddy had acute lymphoblastic leukemia—ALL—a winnable condition at that time. They were on the sixth floor for a long time, and Buddy went into remission.

In the lobby of our floor late one afternoon, a big husky man stalked in with his three equally large sons. They were lumber-jacks, dressed in plaid flannel shirts with blue jeans and heavy boots. The father, red-faced and agitated, paced back and forth. He had been advised that his son's arm would have to be amputated. He told anyone who would listen that the doctors were crazy if they thought they would take his son's arm off. "A man has to work," he said, "and it takes two arms to do it."

His audience said nothing.

After several conferences with the doctors, they gathered their jackets and left. I never saw them again.

Once, Ross and I were asked to talk to a new patient and his family. Mark DeLorenzo, a tall, handsome basketball player, was scheduled for amputation of his arm because of a tumor in his hand. The tumor wasn't considered to be a pediatric form of cancer, and he stayed on another floor. Ross spent several hours with Mark, and the next day I sat with his mother and father while he was in surgery. Ross and Mark were chosen to test the latest improvements in hooks that are used on prosthetic arms.

Mike Murawa had been ill in Toledo, Ohio, for a long time but his condition had been difficult to diagnosis. By the time he reached NIH, more than a year after his problems started, his disease had advanced so far that it couldn't be determined exactly where it had originated. Mike was 19 years old, and Dottie, his mother, had left several younger children at home. Mike suffered terribly for the few months he was there. An air ambulance returned him to Toledo, where he died in a hospital.

Several months after getting established as a member of "the club"on the sixth floor, Ross met Kathy Holloway. Kathy had a tumor in her brain, inoperable, and received chemotherapy and radiation. She lived in nearby Potomac, and occasionally her family invited us out to visit.

On our way to Potomac one day, Ross asked, "What do you think about Kathy, Mom?"

"I can't say that I really know her, Ross. I've never talked much with her. She seems nice and has a nice smile. Her mom is very kind to me—always wanting to know if she can do anything for us since we're so far away from home. I like that. She's very thoughtful."

"We like the same music...We both like animals...We like to travel and go places. We've been to a lot of the same places."

"You and Kathy are older than the others, aren't you?"

"Not really. There's ten or twelve of us who are seniors—and that's just the ones I know about."

"I'm glad you've got a special friend in Kathy. I like her."

"Did you know she had red hair?"

"No, I didn't know that. That's something else you have in common—a couple of hot-tempered redheads."

"She's not hot-tempered at all—just the opposite. She's actually shy, but when you start talking to her, you find out she's real smart. She smiles a lot. I gave her a nickname—'Sunshine'."

"Why doesn't she wear a wig?"

"She does sometimes but not when she's in the hospital. She doesn't like it—says it looks phony. Sometimes she wears a scarf or a funny cap when she's feeling good."

Ross had fun playing with the Holloways' big, rambunctious dog. Pat, Kathy's mother, often told of how Kathy fell and hit her head while on a romp with the dog. Her tumor was discovered a few months later.

I first saw Jesse Lewis, one of the most interesting and inspiring patients with whom I had contact, while standing in the main lobby trying to get on an elevator. I noticed a thin, wiry, black man on crutches. He had only one leg. I watched as he did a twist in time with the jazzy tune he sang. He used his crutch to tap out a beat.

Suddenly, he stopped singing and said, "Oh hell, I forgot my papers!" He pivoted around and took off in an almost run back out through the lobby.

Later in the day, I saw the man again, talking with Andy Tartler, and wondered how he had lost his leg. When I asked Andy, he said he would arrange a meeting, so Jesse came to visit Ross.

"Hey, man," he said, as he hopped athletically into the room. "I'm Jesse Lewis. Andy told me I should meet you."

Ross lifted his heavy eyelids and said, "Hi."

"I'm Elaine—Ross's mother. I asked Andy about you after I saw you downstairs by the elevator. Did you find your papers?"

"Oh, yeah—right where I left them—in the hotel room."

"Where are you staying?"

"Over at United Inn in Bethesda."

Ross had raised his bed and looked at Jesse. "Did you walk all the way back to the hotel?" he asked.

"Yeah, man. It's good for me—can't get too much exercise," he grinned, showing gleaming white teeth.

"You must be in pretty good shape to walk that far on crutches," Ross said.

"When I saw Jesse," I told Ross, "he wasn't walking—he was running."

Jesse laughed. His black skin glistened and his eyes sparkled.

"When did you lose your leg?" Ross asked.

"About seven years ago," he responded. "And then, man, I went through chemotherapy—what a trip!"

"How did you get along with it?" Ross asked.

"Rough, man, really rough. But I survived. You'll survive. You think you won't, but you will. Ever had a thoracotomy?"

"No, and I hope I don't have to."

"That's another story. I've had two. But I made it...I survived. You just gotta have the right attitude—the right frame of mind. Don't let it get you down—you know?"

"I'm trying to have the right attitude," Ross said softly.

"That's all the advice I got for anybody in this scene: Fight cancer with a positive attitude. Don't let it get you down, man. If you do, you're a goner. Don't let it happen."

He rose from his chair and hopped over to the side of Ross's bed. Reaching forth to shake Ross's hand, he said, "You gonna make it, boy. You got what it takes. Keep the faith, brother!"

He pivoted on his crutch and started toward the door.

"Please come back anytime you're in town," I said. "We might be here then. I'd like to keep in touch."

"I'll be around. Still have to come up for my check-ups. I'll find him."

He turned and looked back at Ross. "One more piece of advice, Ross. Endure chemotherapy by smoking marijuana."

"They let you smoke pot here in the hospital?" Ross asked.

"No, they didn't."

"How did you get away with it?"

"I had my ways," Jesse grinned.

"Where did you get it?" I asked, an idea forming in my mind.

"I had my sources," he replied, ending this inquiry as he left the room and hurried toward the elevator.

We never saw Jesse again but kept up with him through the social workers. But I would always remember Jesse Lewis—a bright spot in a world of dark clouds.

The recreational therapy staff made every effort to brighten the atmosphere on the hall. They devised clever themes and decorated the walls with creative and colorful motifs. Once, when entering the hall, I was surprised to see palm trees along with real sand and sea shells. Another time, on a very hot day in the summer, the hall had a decorated Christmas tree and carols were being played on the record player.

However, nothing could actually keep the older patients from knowing the reality of illness and death in the rooms. Because of the sadness and sickness on the sixth floor, combined with the memory of our experiences in the hotels and motels when we first arrived at NIH, I made the decision that every time Ross was discharged, I would find a cheerful and pleasant place to stay. During our tenure in Bethesda we had tried several of the small motels, hotels and inns there, but none could compare with the Bethesda Marriott.

Since Ross felt a little better, he appreciated our new quarters. The doorman, wearing a long red coat and a tall, British-style white hat, opened our car door with a flourish every time I drove up to the entrance.

Within an hour of our arrival, Ross had changed into a bathing suit and tried to slip inconspicuously into the indoor pool. After a few quiet laps around the outer edges, he climbed up the ladder, walked over a few steps and entered the jacuzzi which was already occupied by three men. After a few minutes, he walked up the steps as each of them reached forth to shake his hand.

Later he told me the men were oncologists from the Naval

Hospital, and he was also pleased to let me know they were very interested in his case.

The Marriott staff was extraordinarily kind to us. Once when we checked out expecting to go to Mobile, Ross had a call from NIH telling him not to leave. We had no reservation for another day and the Marriott had no room for us. While we were sitting in the lobby trying to decide what to do, the manager walked by and discovered our dilemma. "Wait a little while," he said. "Let me see what I can do. Go to the Stirrup Lounge—it's Hungry Hour. I'll find you."

While waiting, Ross ate his fill of tacos. In a couple of hours, a bellboy came in and told us our room was ready. A new addition to the hotel was almost finished but not yet ready for guests. Although it was 6:00 in the evening, the manager had the staff hang a door, put up a shower curtain, make the beds, clean the room, and move in a television set, so we had a brand new room to stay in. We never wanted to stay in any other hotel.

It was the middle of March, and in order for Ross to graduate with his class, it was imperative that he get caught up with his studies. In a conference with the oncologists, we learned their recommendation: Return to Mobile soon and begin some of the treatments there.

The next three days of adriamycin were given as an in-patient so that his heart could be monitored. When discharged, he went from room to room on the hall, saying good-bye to staff, patients, and their families.

He went into Kathy's room, where he stayed for an hour. They promised to write each other and exchanged "pre-chemo" snapshots of themselves. Kathy's photo showed her standing on a bridge in London with Big Ben in the background. A bright smile was on her face and her long, shimmering red hair was blowing in the wind.

11

When we returned home on March 12th, I was reminded of how peaceful and still our neighborhood is when compared to the hustle and bustle of Bethesda. After turning out the lights at night, we listen to the familiar sound of a distant train or a dog barking somewhere in the neighborhood. In the mornings, we wake to the singing of birds.

Spring Hill is like a small village. Almost everything needed is within walking distance from our home—churches, schools, library, banks, gift and clothing shops, hair dressers, grocers, drug stores, dry cleaners, and a hardware store.

When our children were little, they knew all the neighbors and their animals. They loved the lady who collected stray cats and they shied away from the ornery man who forbade children to cut a path through his manicured yard.

Ross was four years old when we moved into our house. He missed his former playmates and was constantly seeking attention with some exciting discovery or plan. Since animals often wandered around our neighborhood at night—possums, raccoons, rabbits, and turtles—he planned a sanctuary in our back yard. He drew a picture of an aviary he wanted to build, with fruit trees for the birds. A fountain was part of his plan so the animals and birds would always have water.

His favorite time—the evening meal—was when he listened to Mary's and Scott's events of the day and tried to match their stories with his activities. He wanted to stay up at night as late as they did, and was usually the last one in the family to go to sleep. It was important to him that the family be together, everyone in his or her place.

Before Mary reached the teen years, Scott went to first grade and Ross started playschool. Since we lived two blocks from the school, our house became a good stopping place for other children to play. Those were the happy years.

∾

Mobile begins to put its best face forward during the month of March. The city is glorious with azaleas, dogwood, bridal wreath, wisteria, and Japanese magnolias. All the colors create a spectacle of awesome splendor. It was the right time to be home.

For the first two weeks, Ross attempted school, but, when he learned how far behind he was, he became discouraged. His counselor advised him to drop all subjects except those necessary to graduate. They allowed him to recycle some good 11th grade research papers and assigned some special condensed studies.

Most of his classmates had applied to various colleges and many had already received their acceptances. The UMS faculty recommended that he apply to a small college, preferably nearby.

Since Spring Hill College had an enrollment of about 1,000 students, and since it was only two blocks from our home, there was no good reason to look elsewhere. The UMS counselor contacted the Admissions Office at Spring Hill and explained Ross's circumstances.

Ross knew the campus very well, having played there for many years. He began to look at it from a different perspective. As he drove us across the campus, he scanned the buildings and grounds as if seeing them for the first time. He parked the car near the Administration Building and we walked down the hill under a canopied walkway. Although he had insisted I go with him, when we reached the door, he asked me to wait outside. "I'll call you if I need you," he said.

He entered the office, and I wandered around the campus. Spring Hill College is the oldest college in the State of Alabama. Founded by the Jesuits, it also has the reputation of being a very difficult school. Many of its buildings are pre-Civil War. Sprawling, old oaks with Spanish moss, dogwood trees, camellia and azalea bushes line the winding, narrow streets on top of what is believed to be the actual crest known as Spring Hill.

Across a narrow street, I could see Mobile's skyline several miles away. On a hill which sloped toward Mirror Lake, a grounds-keeper raked leaves inside a white picket fence around a very old cemetery where white crosses marked the graves of priests. As I sat on a bench under the oak trees with their bright green buds, I listened to a piano lesson being given in a classroom nearby. The music echoed between the buildings.

In a few minutes, I saw Ross waving in my direction. He walked briskly down the hill and said, "They said they'd be glad to consider me. I'm not too far behind and they said I could get some tutoring if I need it."

"The big question now is whether you want to go here."

"No, that's not it. I do want to go here. The big question is how much it costs. It's real expensive, Mom."

"I've heard that it is. We'll have to talk to your dad about it. Let's don't bring it up to him right now. He has a lot of things on his mind, and he's planning to fly to Washington to drive my car back home. Maybe we can work something out. I plan to find another job as soon as you finish your treatments."

"There might be some kind of scholarships. Maybe I could get a student loan. I'd like to live on campus someday but that can wait. I hope they'll accept me."

It was a big boost to his morale later in the week when he learned he had been accepted.

This news motivated Ross to try to get caught up enough to graduate. It was frustrating because there were days when he felt so ill that he couldn't go to class. Also, looming ahead for the coming week was another treatment of chemotherapy.

Adriamycin, followed immediately by the one remaining drug which had not yet been given, cis platin, was on the agenda.

While his friends were in school, Ross was lonely. He missed our dog which had been given to friends who had a farm because the free-spirited animal couldn't adapt to a fenced-in yard. He asked if we could get another dog.

We visited the city pound, but nothing interested him that day. We browsed around in a pet store. He spoke of a dog he had met briefly during the summer when he was in Washington taking care of Mary. He and Mary were on a picnic at a lake when a big, friendly white dog came over to play. He didn't know the name of the breed. In the pet shop, he spied a booklet in the rack with a picture of the dog on the front of it.

"That's it!" he said. "It's a Samoyed."

We called several veterinarians, and when the word got around that Ross wanted a Samoyed, we found a puppy for sale in Mobile.

The owner led us into her kitchen, and there on the floor was a most unusual, beautiful little puppy. Ross squatted on the floor and snapped his fingers. The snow-white, long-haired little puppy perked up his ears, ambled over, and licked his hand. After we carried him to our car, he never seemed to doubt that he belonged to Ross. Ross named him "Prince Rocky," but a better name might have been "Luke"—the Great Physician.

Rocky chewed the legs of chairs and the corners of rugs. He dug holes in the yard, then raced through the house with his white fur covered with black dirt. The white coat shed all over everything. But he never left Ross's side. He was a joy.

12

Ross walked into the kitchen one day and said, "Mom, could you sit down a minute? I need to talk to you about something."

I pulled out a chair and sat across from him. "What's up?"

"You know I've got cis platin coming up next week. What do you think about me smoking marijuana?"

"You mean in the hospital? I doubt if they'll allow it. But I don't care if you want to try it. Anything that will help is fine with me. You're remembering Jesse Lewis, aren't you?"

"He's not the only one, Mom. Some of the other patients said they tried it, too."

"Let's talk to Dr. Clarkson about it."

"I'm not talking to Dr. Clarkson about it. He'd probably say no. I don't care what he says. I want to try it."

I overruled him, and on Monday, I went with him to Dr. Clarkson's office when he went for blood work and to discuss his coming treatment. Ross brought up the subject of smoking marijuana in an effort to relieve the nausea. He told the doctor of different things he had tried while at NIH, and though one anti-emetic drug had been found which sometimes helped when taking methotrexate, nothing had worked with BCD. The next scheduled treatment, adriamycin, hadn't caused nausea when given by itself, but also coming up was the tough one—cis platin.

Ross knew from other patients and the protocol sheet that this was the worst one of all.

"I have no objection to your trying marijuana," Dr. Clarkson said. "But with cis platin, I doubt it will do any good."

"I'd still like to try it."

"Okay. I'll clear it with the officials at the Mobile Infirmary, but don't say anything about it to anyone and keep the room door closed when you're smoking it."

Ross turned his head and looked at me.

I shrugged my shoulders and said, "Okay with me."

Dr. Clarkson added, "Ross, in the past I could have provided the marijuana for you because I could get it from the sheriff's office. But all that has changed now, so I have no way to get it. You'll have to provide it yourself."

The wheels started turning in my thoughts.

Dr. Clarkson gave Ross a prescription for the drug THC, a derivative of marijuana, and told him to go to the University of South Alabama Medical Center Pharmacy to get it filled—the only place in Mobile where it could be purchased. He instructed him to start taking the pills several hours before admission to the hospital. We drove to the USAMC pharmacy and purchased the THC.

"What about the pot?" Ross asked.

"I'll make the purchase of the marijuana, Ross," I said, remembering how he'd suffered in previous treatments. "Don't worry, I'll get it."

"You? You've got be kidding!" he laughed. "Really, Mom, what do you know about pot? You wouldn't know it if you saw it. Let me handle it."

"No, I'll take care of it," I told him, hoping he couldn't tell from my expression that he was absolutely right.

That evening, we told Bill of the plan and he hit the ceiling. There was no way we were going to do this. We endured his litany of reasons why it could not be done: It was immoral, illegal, stupid, and ridiculous.

Ross and I listened.

Later, when Bill left, Ross and I, the foolish and reckless co-conspirators, discussed how he would actually smoke it, since his right hand would be immobile. He concluded that he needed a water pipe and he knew of a "head" shop in the mall where he could get one. It was news to me that a store existed in Mobile that specialized in such equipment. I gave him the money for it.

Among the many young people I knew who had the reputation of using marijuana, I couldn't get up the nerve to call one and say, "How about selling me some pot?" Then I remembered a good friend who had grown up through the sixties during the turbulent times and fancied himself to be a man-of-the-world during that era. Although he lived away from Mobile, I called him and explained my dilemma.

"Lordy, lordy, I gave up that life years ago," he said.

"I know you did, but I thought you could refresh your memory enough to tell me how to go about this."

"Let me think about it for awhile. I'll be in touch."

The next day, he called back. "Don't ask me any questions. Just follow these instructions and do what I say."

I apologized for putting him in this position.

"It's okay, don't worry about it. I'm completely out of touch with that world and it took longer than I thought it would. But everything is arranged now, so don't worry about it."

"I appreciate the trouble you've gone to," I offered, feeling like part of a mysterious intrigue.

"Forget it—no problem," he said. "Tomorrow morning, first thing when you get up, go to your back door and there will be a package there."

I waited for his next instructions. He was silent.

"Is that all? Is this dangerous? Will someone get in trouble? Have you told anyone else about this?"

"Remember, I told you to ask me no questions," he said before saying good-bye.

I began to get nervous. Ross came in later with the water pipe. It was somewhat attractive and I wondered if it could be used for something else, something legal. We put it together and he showed me how it worked. I briefly wondered how he knew so much about it, but I let the thought pass and reassured him that I would take care of the other purchase. Before Bill came home, we hid the water pipe.

Early the next morning, I hurried down the stairs and went straight to the back door. There, on the back step, I saw a small plastic sandwich bag with a bit of what appeared to be dried, crumbled oregano. Is this all? I thought, remembering the quoted cost. Quickly, I put the bag in my robe pocket and started preparing breakfast. Ross left for school, Bill left for work, and I began to gather Ross's hospital clothes.

At noon, Ross came home from school, got out of his uniform, and took the first THC pill. With a silly grin on his face, we drove to Dr. Clarkson's office for hospital orders and Ross turned over his chemotherapy drugs which he had brought from NIH. Dr. Clarkson reviewed his protocol, wrote out the orders, and we proceeded to the hospital for his admission to the Mobile Infirmary—the first one for chemotherapy.

We finally reached his room a few minutes after 4:00 that afternoon and were in awe of the large, private space. Soon someone brought a cot for me. I hadn't requested one and wondered what it was for.

The halls seemed empty compared to NIH. Ross strolled around, getting his bearings and introducing himself to anyone he could find. Remembering the cheerful chatter on the sixth floor at NIH, the Infirmary personnel seemed somber and serious. Ross missed the special attention he got at NIH.

His nurse, a middle-aged woman with a grim face, came in to start prehydration. Without talking, she strapped his right arm and hand stiffly to a board and poked around until she had the needle inserted.

"What's my schedule?" Ross asked. "Do you know when the drugs will be started?"

The nurse said, "I'm waiting for the pharmacy to bring the mixture up. We'll give the adriamicin first. After it's finished, we wait for two hours, then we start the cis platin."

A long night loomed before us. After the nurse left the room, I unpacked the water pipe and hid it in the bathroom.

Bill arrived and discovered it. He pulled himself up to full height and announced, "I want you both to know, and I'll go on record, that I oppose the use of illegal drugs, no matter what the circumstances! Do you understand what I'm saying?"

"I understand. Anything else?" I asked.

"That's all I have to say."

Ross and I looked at each other—but for just a moment—until our unspoken decision was reached. He said, "Mom, you stand with your back to the door and don't let anyone come in."

I took my position.

"Dad, you'll have to light the pipe and hold it for me."

With tight lips, Bill looked at me with fire in his eyes. Then he rolled his eyes upward, looked up at the ceiling for a full minute, then glared at me again. Finally, he took a deep breath and twisted his face into a tight frown. He picked up the water pipe, lit the wick, leaned back and stretched out his arms to hold the pipe to Ross as though distancing himself as far as possible from the act. The sweet smell filled the room.

We hid the pipe in the bathroom before the nurse returned.

It took one hour for the adriamycin to go through the needle, and though the nurse said nothing, her expression of repugnance revealed that she knew what had been going on in the room. When she left, we re-lit the pipe, and again Bill held it.

At 11:00 p.m., the cis platin was started, and Ross seemed to fare well. Maybe his "premed of choice" was helping.

But it didn't last. Vomiting started at 3:00 a.m. The bed shook as he started trembling violently with chills. I pushed the call button and a different nurse came in.

"Take his temperature," I said, while holding Ross's shoulders up so his head was over the basin.

"I took it not long ago. It was normal," she said.

"Please take it again," I said, panic rising in my voice.

"Don't get upset, Mrs. Phelps. It's not necessary to take it this soon."

"Then give me the thermometer. Now!" I demanded. "And get the head nurse in here, right now!"

She left the room and in a few minutes came back with a breathless RN who had run from another wing on the floor. She popped the thermometer in Ross's mouth in between heaves and vomiting. I wondered if his insides were dissolving.

The thermometer registered 102 degrees. It had climbed to that point in less than an hour.

"Call Dr. Clarkson, please," I said.

"Yes ma'am," the nurse replied as she walked out the door.

Within minutes, Dr. Clarkson came in and gave instructions for emergency procedures to slow the rising temperature. He ordered an antibiotic IV, and made the decision then and there that the next dose of cis platin would be cut in half.

The retching slowed about daylight the following morning and finally ended around 10:00 a.m. The nauseous feeling continued.

I dreaded having to admit to Bill that the marijuana hadn't worked.

Later in the morning, when Ross finished his last nausea upheaval, his pale skin emphasized the black shadows under his eyes. His bald scalp was a gray, pasty color. He wore a white tee shirt and white gym shorts—his standard hospital wardrobe of choice. He looked like a ghost.

My face hadn't been washed and my hair hadn't been combed. I flopped down in a chair with my legs stretched out in front of me, closed my eyes, and drifted off to sleep.

There was a soft tap on the door. I had failed to remember that Ross would have visitors in the hospital in Mobile.

Our minister entered the room, his eyes moving from Ross to me. He mumbled something, and, with tears in his eyes, he turned and hurried out.

I could have used a word from the Lord. But what could a minister say, when even God Himself was silent.

Covering my face and eyes with my hands in an attempt to hold back the tears, my shoulders started shaking. But instead of crying, I started a quiet, uncontrollable laughter.

"What's funny?" Ross mumbled, his eyes half closed.

"Nothing, honey...nothing." I wiped my eyes and blew my nose as the deep giggles continued to spill out.

"What did he say?"

"I don't know. Something about courage, I think. Go on to sleep if you can."

"What's funny about that?"

"It's not funny, Ross. At least, he didn't intend it to be funny."

"Why are you laughing? What's wrong with you?"

"I'm okay," I said as I rose from the chair. "I'll be back in a minute. I'm going to get a drink of water. Now I've got hiccups. Try to go on to sleep."

As I slowly walked along the hall, the realization came that I had placed ministers on that same pedestal where some doctors were stationed and had expected a more-than-human response.

Some ministers who visited Ross eased quietly into the room and left a calling card on his bedside table. Others volunteered prayer and Bible reading. Sometimes they talked about the weather, the traffic, or current events.

Once, when Ross had school visitors standing around his bed, a minister came in with a great flurry of greeting, hugging me tightly, whirling around while lifting his face to the ceiling and quickly praying for God's blessing. He dramatically intoned his plea and finished his prayer before Ross and his visitors realized he'd been praying.

During Ross's year of treatment, he was exposed to many types of non-religious and religious beliefs—from the most fundamental Christian practices, both Protestant and Catholic, to Orthodox Jewish tenets. A couple of times I had a problem with that. It bothered me when a relative or visitor of a roommate would be evangelical in presenting their beliefs to the captive audience on the other side of the curtain. Ross said he didn't mind. He listened attentively and didn't debate. He reminded me that people do the best they can when trying to make sense out of situations like ours.

Ross and I would have been very hurt and disappointed if our ministers hadn't called on us. Someday, I thought, I might try to write a book about how *not* to visit a patient in cancer treatment. But I couldn't think of a single line to put in it.

When I reentered Ross's room, he appeared to be sleeping. Later that afternoon, I again took out the water pipe. I had completely lost faith in it doing any good, but Ross wanted to try again. At that moment, I would have given him anything he asked for.

After a few whiffs on the pipe, this time with me lighting and holding the contraption and not caring who saw it, the nausea eased and he didn't heave again. He fell into a peaceful sleep which continued all night.

The conclusion I reached was that marijuana could be very effective for tension and for keeping down queasy feelings. In the presence of violent nausea, it was worthless.

The next day, Good Friday, he went home. After cis platin, no further treatments could be given for at least three weeks.

13

April, 1983

On Saturday, our New Orleans relatives stopped by and Ross's cousins spent the night with us while their mother Dorothy proceeded on to the country, near Lucedale, for Jean and Bud Persons' annual Easter family reunion.

We joined them on Sunday for the gathering of our clan. Mary couldn't make it all the way from Washington, and Ross's Aunt Hilda and Uncle Jack Heflin lived in California—too far away to make a brief trip south. But Joe and Vilma, their children and grandchildren, my step-mother, my half-sister, Ann Rollins and her husband Lloyd, my half-brother, Nevon Johnston, and their families joined the festivities by the fish pond, trying their hand in what we called "The Persons' Fishing Rodeo."

A sumptuous meal awaited us at the Persons' home. Their property was in the woods about a mile off the county road and provided a perfect spot for children to play, hide Easter eggs, and walk in the woods picking wild flowers. Impromptu games of team frisbee and touch football were vigorously pursued.

Ross learned that, after casting the fishing line out with his right hand and adjusting the position of the hook on his prosthesis, he could turn the reel using the device. He had found one sport he could do—a boost to his spirit. He had plenty of help tying lures and untangling lines from the Persons' young sons, Russell and Tosh, who cheered him on.

After a couple of hours of fishing, he announced that he had to leave in order to join his senior classmates on their annual spend-the-night party at Dauphin Island. Monday would be "senior skip-day." He waited until surrounded by allies—uncles, aunts and cousins—before mentioning this plan to me.

The following Saturday was senior prom night, and, at the last minute, Ross found a date with a pretty girl—a younger sister of one of his classmates. He managed to rent a tux, order a corsage, and make plans to double-date with another senior. His tux fit nicely and he seemed satisfied. Then he put on his dark brown suede hat and his white sneakers. He left in high spirits, with a smile on his face.

The parents of the seniors were invited to watch the call-outs. The junior class was responsible for putting on the prom, which, when translated, meant the mothers of the junior boys had done most of the work. The club where the dance was held was decorated in a posh jungle theme—lush greenery with colorful tropical birds in wicker cages. It was filled with twittering teenagers, constantly moving, calling out to each other above the loud music.

As we watched the call-outs, I saw that several of Ross's friends also had on hats and white sneakers with their tux.

During the following week, Ross bought a new rod and reel, and he and his classmate and friend, Lawrence Sims, returned to the Persons' pond after school. They hauled in a record catch of trout which they proudly spread out on the patio, then photographed.

On another trip, I went with him back to the pond and he caught a huge large-mouthed bass, which thrilled him. His Aunt Jean took the fish to a taxidermist and had it mounted on a wooden plaque.

As we were driving home, I told him that I had recently had a telephone call from Mike Murawa's mother. Ross knew that Mike had died two weeks before. Dottie and Mike's father, Chuck, were going on a trip to Florida and had decided to detour to Mobile to visit us.

I remembered the day the Murawas left the sixth floor of NIH. Dottie—a petite lady with a set, determined smile—handed out long-stemmed red roses to each of the nurses while Mike's gurney and entourage waited for the elevator with all the equipment for sustaining his life. A dedicated Catholic family with several priests and nuns among their relatives, heaven had been stormed with prayers for Mike.

Thinking about the Murawas' planned visit, I discussed the possibility of having a special mass said for Mike with Father Bobby Rimes at Spring Hill College. He suggested that we use the tiny historic chapel on campus.

Both Catholic and Protestant friends attended. Ross was excused from school in time to be there at 2:00. With Chuck Murawa assisting at the altar, Father Rimes gave an inspiring and comforting message.

Ross remained silent about the Murawas' visit. I reminded him that Mike didn't have an early diagnosis.

School, playing with Rocky, being tutored by his friend Jim, and fishing at the Persons', occupied all Ross's free time. His blood counts were too low for that week's scheduled treatment of adriamycin and cis platin. The postponement meant he could go to another prom—this time sponsored by Wright's School for Girls—the companion of UMS Prep School for Boys. His temperature had begun to climb slightly, but he planned to double-date with Jim, who promised to bring him home promptly if needed.

Jim arrived at our house to pick Ross up dressed in full regalia of formal wear. Six feet tall and still growing, Jim was a handsome young man who could have served as a model for his outfit—dark brown hair, neatly combed; big brown eyes alert and sparkling. I rarely saw him when he didn't have a sincere smile.

"As usual, Jim, he's not ready. His dad is up there with him trying to get all the pieces together and the buttons in place. I'm sorry you always have to wait for him."

"No problem, Mrs. Phelps. I don't mind."

"You sure put up with a lot from him, Jim," I said as I looked him squarely in the eye.

He returned my gaze. "I'd do anything in the world for him, Mrs. Phelps. He's been the best friend I've ever had."

"He feels the same way about you. You have been so faithful. I know how busy you are."

"He's worth it. Things like this shouldn't happen to guys like Ross. He's one of the good guys. He's different."

"What do you mean?"

He lowered his eyes and tilted his head, not looking at me. "I don't know—I don't know how to describe it, but he's got certain things about him. He cares about people, you know? I mean—really cares. He's understanding. He doesn't bad-mouth people. He doesn't try to pretend he's something he's not. He's just...Ross...."

I said to Jim, "It means a lot to Ross and me to know that you and Kit White are always available when he needs you. When I hear a soft knock on the door, I can guess that it's Kit outside. Like you, he's a faithful friend. I know Ross has called both of you a lot from NIH, and sometimes those calls must have been painful for you."

"It's all right, Mrs. Phelps. I believe Ross is going to make it."

May, 1983

The following Sunday, Ross left in the morning, drove to the Gulf alone and stayed the entire day. It was May, eight months from diagnosis and I had been told that it could take several months for the reality of the whole picture to be grasped. For more than three weeks, there had been no chemotherapy and he could think clearer thoughts. He had witnessed the heroic efforts on the part of the medical team for Mike Murawa and others who didn't respond.

Tuesday after school, he and I returned to the fish pond in the country. It was a beautiful spring afternoon. As Ross drove along the wooded back roads, he speculated and philosophized about life, death, and the state of humanity in general. He posed questions, then answered as if he were thinking out loud. When we reached Jean's house, he decided to go for a walk in the woods before he started fishing.

Jean and I sat outside under an oak and breathed in the newness of the young greening of the trees, grass and shrubbery.

"What's going on with Lana Dungan?" I asked.

"I was hoping you wouldn't ask," she said.

"She's not doing well?"

"I've heard that she's not. I don't know any details."

"These kids will surprise you. They can be so terribly ill, then go into remission."

"I hope you're right. She's fought so hard for so long."

"Will you let me know when you hear anything else from her?"

"Okay. Let's walk down to the pond."

The next day when Ross was admitted to the Mobile Infirmary for the scheduled round of treatment, he again took the THC pills and I packed the water pipe.

That night, a young, chatty, officious nurse came in to start the IV. She authoritatively explained chemotherapy treatment to Ross as if he had never heard of it before. Although Ross had told her that there were no good veins in certain areas, she insisted on trying in those spots anyway.

Ross clenched his teeth as beads of sweat formed above his lip. He frowned as he watched her continue to stick him with the needle. The more she failed, the more tense he became.

"Why don't you just leave it alone for awhile?" he asked. "Maybe if you come back later, it'll be okay."

She brushed her long hair out of her face and said, "I can't wait because you have to be prehydrated and you need to get started." She continued to probe, again and again.

Ross glared at me.

I asked, "Could you get someone else to come in and try—someone who already knows how difficult his veins are?"

"No, no, I can find one," she said, as she bent over and stuck the needle into his arm again.

"Stop it! No more!" Ross yelled, as he jerked his arm away and started to cry.

"Leave him alone! Please, please leave him alone," I said.

"Well, what do you suggest I do? I've got to start it," she said, with exasperation.

"I don't care what you do," said Ross. "Just get out and leave me alone!"

She haughtily left the room for a few minutes and then returned to the door. "Can I try again now, Mr. Phelps?" she called to him with a feigned cheerfulness.

"No! Get out of my room!" he shouted.

"Well, I'm going to have to call the doctor and tell him that you refused to let me start prehydration."

"I don't care what you do, or who you call. Just leave me alone!"

I took out the water pipe, lit it, and held it to him.

In a few minutes, the phone rang. It was Dr. Meshad, Dr. Clarkson's partner, who was on call. He talked with Ross for a few minutes, then Ross handed the phone to me.

"I told the nurses to leave him alone," he said. "They're not to go in his room except to check his vital signs unless he calls."

"Thank you," I said. And thank God, I thought as I hung up the phone.

After sitting quietly for a few minutes, I left Ross in the darkened room and walked to the end of the hall where I stood and stared out the window toward the sprawling parking lot in front of the hospital. All around us on the hall were very sick people. Maybe I should have tried to coax Ross into letting the nurse try to get the IV started.

The grapevine on the hall had informed all the nurses about

the scene in Ross's room. Some of them already knew of my temper from the night his fever spiked, and I suspected all of them knew about the marijuana. I avoided their eyes as I slowly walked back toward the room, my head bowed low and my arms folded.

I heard footsteps beside me which matched my own, and felt an arm being gently placed around my shoulder. I turned my head and looked into the eyes of a doctor I knew. We didn't speak. When we arrived at Ross's door, I stopped.

"I know this is tough," he said.

"Yes, it is."

He squeezed my hand and continued along the hall.

Just a few years before, he had lost his 18-year-old son in an automobile accident. I had heard that he and his wife had received this news over the telephone during the night.

Instead of going into Ross's room, I sauntered to the other end of the hall, still staring at the floor. I thought of another doctor I had seen in the halls of the hospital who had recently lost his son to bone cancer. The boy was a couple of years older than Ross and they had many mutual friends. When he died, about six weeks after Ross was diagnosed with a similar disease, their friends were stunned. They lived not far from us in Spring Hill and the boy had been a patient at NIH.

Several of our friends had experienced tragedies with their children. I remembered Helen and Art Wells of our church who had lost Melanie, their teenage daughter, to leukemia more than ten years before. The Marsh's daughter, Stephanie, had died of osteosarcoma not long after moving to Mobile and joining our church. Gary Bradshaw, 18-year-old son of close friends, Fred and Kaye, had died as the result of an automobile accident on an icy street in Connecticut on New Year's Eve just a few years before. Three years prior, Paige Faddis, 23-year-old son of our good friends Anne and Ed, had been in a minor automobile accident. Twenty-four hours later, he slipped into a coma, and when awakened a few days later, was a quadriplegic.

I thought of mothers who had seen their sons leave for war in a foreign country. Some of their sons never returned, and of those who did, many were scarred, emotionally and physically. Some even lost limbs. There were those whose children had been deeply involved in drugs—some who went to jail and even on to prison. I remembered seeing a new patient being brought into the Clinic at NIH handcuffed between two men. He appeared to be just a little older than Ross. There were those I didn't know but only read about in the newspapers, who were in prison on death row. That's some mother's son, I thought.

I had lived naively, assuming that my family would be exempt from deep suffering.

After slowly walking back and forth in the hall, lost in these thoughts, I returned to Ross's room and sat quietly in the dark. He finally fell asleep and I opened the little cot and lay there pondering the meaning of all of this.

Early Saturday morning, Dr. Meshad arrived and sat by the bed, leaning forward, close to Ross's head. Though Dr. Meshad usually cracked jokes and spouted witticisms, he started speaking softly but seriously to Ross.

I left the room and when I returned a few minutes later, a nurse stood by Dr. Meshad and the IV was in operation.

"What happened?" I asked. "Looks like everything is all right this morning."

"Oh, no problem," Dr. Meshad said. "I just warned Ross if he didn't behave himself, I would put the chemo up his nose."

Ross chuckled as I followed Dr. Meshad out the door.

"Now, tell me what really happened," I said.

He explained a simple logic: The more tense a patient becomes, the tighter the veins and blood vessels constrict.

I wondered if the knowledgeable nurse from the previous evening had missed class the day that was taught.

Adriamycin was finished at noon, and, an hour later, cis platin was started. Four hours into the cis platin dosage, the vomiting began and continued almost constantly until midnight.

When he was discharged on Sunday, his friends gathered around. They gave Rocky a bath and kept Ross company for the rest of the day. He made it to school the next morning but had to return home because of nausea. He threw up all afternoon.

Other problems arose which could not be ignored. Cramps were occurring all over his body—in his neck, shoulders, chest, stomach, and legs. Through urine analysis, it was learned that his body was being depleted of magnesium, a necessary mineral. The Informed Consent document had stated that cis platin could cause kidney damage, and if severe, might not be reversible. Often the kidneys failed to filter and retain essential minerals or trace elements. Magnesium tablets were prescribed to be taken daily. When the dosage reached 30 tablets a day, the cramps subsided.

On Thursday, while at school, he suffered a blackout and, although he recovered quickly, it frightened him. The next day he came home when he felt another attack coming on. Nothing definite was found by Dr. Clarkson to explain the blackouts. He suspected it might be caused by fluctuating blood pressure. By this time, we believed that chemotherapy could cause anything.

He struggled to school the next week and took his last exam on Wednesday. Slowly, he began to feel better, and received a clear report on chest X-rays from the Mobile Infirmary.

School was now behind him and the pressure had eased.

14

May, 1983

On Baccalaureate Sunday, Bill and I sat in the auditorium as the seniors filed in wearing their school uniforms—gray pants, navy blazers, blue shirts with striped ties. I craned my neck but couldn't spot Ross.

Then the leaders of the service marched in along with the students who were participating, and they all went up on the stage. There was Ross—without his hat. He kept his eyes glued to the floor. Immediately before they walked down the aisle, the headmaster had told him to take the hat off because it wouldn't be appropriate to wear in a Baccalaureate service.

Our minister at Spring Hill Presbyterian Church, Dr. Vernon Hunter, delivered the address. Not long into his sermon, while speaking of courage, spirit, and valor, he pointed to Ross as an example. Ross sat there with his bald head bowed, looking at the floor. After the sermon was finished, Ross rose and walked to the podium to deliver the student prayer. I don't think anyone heard what he said.

On graduation night the auditorium was packed with friends and relatives. In caps and gowns, the seniors marched down the aisle to the strains of *Pomp and Circumstance*. Thank God for mortarboards.

Prior to handing out the diplomas, the headmaster presented awards. He called Ross to come on stage. He handed him the Headmaster's Award for Courage. Before he finished making the presentation speech, his voice broke and he had to turn his head away in order to wipe his eyes. Ross received a long standing ovation.

A reception "under the oaks" and tossing of caps in the air climaxed the evening. Ross quickly put on the brown hat before he received many hugs and handshakes.

Thursday, the seniors left on an excursion to New Orleans and returned the next morning at 6:00 a.m. Ross fell in bed and slept until the middle of the afternoon, when all of us—Bill, Scott, Ross, Rocky and I—went to the beach.

Rocky skipped up and down the beach, barking at the noise of the breakers. As the waves crashed on the shore, he skittered back to Scott and Ross, then chased again as they pulled back into the ocean. When the boys entered the edge of the water, Rocky growled and snapped at the waves as if he was protecting them from a threat.

Late Saturday afternoon, Jim and Kit came over, along with two of Scott's friends. They stayed outside on a pier and talked, their laughter drifting up to the house. Scott had taken his guitar, and he strummed soft melodies which seemed to be in tune with the music of the waves of the receding tide.

"What's with those guys?" I asked Bill. "They seem so quiet—most unusual."

"I don't know. What do you mean?" he asked, as he turned from the television.

"I guess I expected some rough-house—their usual horsing around," I said.

"They're probably worn out from all the partying."

"Is it possible that maybe they're growing up?"

"They're not boys anymore," Bill said as he looked toward the horizon.

That night, under a full moon, they sailed until 3:00 a.m., exploring the inlets of Perdido Bay. Little islands away from traffic and car lights gave an undisturbed view of the heavens.

On Sunday, Ross didn't want to leave, so Bill, Scott and Rocky went home and he and I stayed another night in the cooling breeze and the gentle sounds of the ocean waves.

Monday morning, we returned home to reality: BCD at the Mobile Infirmary.

"What about the water pipe?" I asked. "Are you going to try it again?"

"I guess not. It hasn't done any good so far."

"Let's leave it at home. We have enough to keep up with. If you change your mind, maybe your dad will bring it."

"Are you kidding? That will never happen," he said, as he shook his head and smiled.

When we reached his room, an attractive, well-groomed nurse came in, reached for Ross's hand and introduced herself. She spoke quietly to him about her own son who she said was about Ross's age. With a smile on her face and a twinkle in her eyes, she moved slowly yet efficiently, and promptly found a vein to start the prehydration. The drugs were pushed through the needle as she sat by the bed, making light conversation while she worked. She didn't falter when a fire alarm rang. She remained calmly at Ross's side, reassuring him that it was only a drill.

I took out my notebook and wrote down her name.

She finished giving the drugs at 6:00 p.m. Vomiting started at 8:30 p.m. and continued every five minutes until midnight. His nurse kept close watch until the shift changed at 11:00. The vomiting slowed but continued until daylight.

The next day, the same nurse was on duty when the drugs were started again at noon. After the first one was finished, the needle stopped working. A tall and lanky male technician came in to assist in getting it working again without having to reinsert the needle. Another name was entered in my notebook.

They were finished at 3:30 p.m. and the vomiting began immediately and continued wracking his body until after midnight. This round broke all previous records for the number of times he had to be lifted over the emesis basins.

He was discharged the next day. On Sunday, Jim came to get him and took him on a long drive. On Monday, another friend, M. K. Harless, took him to the Gulf. Ross called from the

Harless family's place and said they had decided to spend the night. M. K. had taken him out in a boat and convinced him that he could still water ski.

When he returned home the next day, pale and exhausted, he had a little sparkle in his eyes.

"Have a good time?" I asked.

"Great. But my legs are so weak. I'm still shaking. I fell about fifty times, but M. K. wouldn't let me quit. He brought the boat around every time I fell and yelled at me to grab the rope. Then he would take off again, and I would fall again. Then he'd come back."

"I don't know how you did it. It makes me weak just thinking about it."

"I don't know either. But you know M. K.—when he makes up his mind, he's determined."

"Yes. 'Wild and Wooly' M. K. Wild horses can't hold him."

"It took me a long time to get my balance. I had to learn how to ski all over again."

"I've seen you ski before holding on with just one hand."

"True, but I'm not strong now. I'm really out of shape—the muscles in my legs have gone to pot. But the biggest problem is the balance. My left shoulder is smaller and my whole weight and balance has shifted. I've gotten used to it but it sure interfered with skiing."

"But now you can ski. Will M. K. take you back again?"

"As soon as I get over this trip. I've got to get my legs in shape. When I finally got up, M. K. pulled me all over Perdido Bay. He revved up the motor, circled around—waving to everybody he saw."

"M. K. is so reckless—wild and reckless," I said.

"Don't criticize him, Mom. He's my friend."

June had arrived—the time when Mobile families take the one-hour drive to Gulf Shores for a vacation in the sun, sand, and blue-green waters of the Gulf of Mexico.

Because Ross was in chemotherapy treatment, he had to avoid

the sun. The danger of infection when his blood counts were low made the risks too great. Other things loomed ahead for him. It was time to return to NIH for bone scans, CT scans, tomograms, X-rays, and another round of methotrexate.

He spent the night before we left at a hotel with Don Mosley, another high school friend. Someone was staging a graduation party. When he returned home at 9:00 a.m., I met him at the door and propelled him to the car. We barely made our flight.

15

June, 1983

Bill had driven my car back to Mobile in March, so Mary met us at Dulles Airport with a new friend's automobile. Frank Lambert, Mary's new romantic interest, had lent the car to us with the stipulation that I had to do all the driving. Since we were accustomed to small, compact cars, the big sedan was a challenge.

Ross had been up all night at the hotel in Mobile, so he fell asleep before we reached Bethesda. His first appointment at NIH the following morning at 9:00 was for injection of dye into his veins in preparation for the bone scan at noon. Following the injection, the schedule called for a tomogram, then chest and arm X-rays, then a CT scan, and finally, the bone scan.

The bone scan takes more than an hour and the technicians permitted me to sit in the darkened room with Ross. I picked up a magazine and sat near the door in the light of the hallway.

The machine moved slowly over Ross's head, and I occasionally glanced at the screen, watching his skeleton appear. Since he had to lay flat on his back, perfectly still, he couldn't see the screen as clearly as I could. He didn't have to take his prosthesis off, and was fully dressed as he lay on the narrow table. It had become routine.

The machine softly clicked and moved down his body. I

watched the screen as it scanned slowly over his left elbow and the abrupt end of his arm. Ross squinted his eyes and frowned, trying to see the screen from his position.

Suddenly, a bright light appeared on his right wrist, exactly as it had been seen on the left one when he had the first scan done the previous September. I stared in disbelief, but said nothing to him.

"Mom, what's that on my arm?"

"I don't know. Just be very still."

"Can you see something? Is that my prosthesis making that shiny spot?"

I rose and took a few steps nearer the screen.

"Which arm is that on, Mom? Tell me what you see."

"I don't know, Ross. Let me find the technician."

Terrified, I moved out into the hall and quickly walked toward the desk. The technician followed me back toward the scanning area when she saw the expression on my face. After taking a look at the screen, she whirled out the door and along the hall, where she disappeared into an office. Several other people crowded into the scanning room in the semi-darkness.

"Get his record," someone said.

They all stood, transfixed.

"I said, get his record—now!" the voice repeated.

One by one, they left the room and went around the corner.

Ross remained frozen as the machine continued to click on its path down his body. Time stood still.

Someone came in and asked, "Ross, when you got your dye injection this morning, where did they stick you?"

"In my right wrist," he said.

Another conference was held at the end of the hall with more checking of the morning record. At last, a technician came in and said, "Relax, Ross. We think we know the answer. When you got your injection this morning, the vein probably collapsed and the dye 'puddled' in your wrist. You just have a big glob of dye in that spot."

After catching my breath, I moved near Ross's head and saw that his shirt was soaking wet. His forehead was icy cold.

The next morning, after admission to the hospital and arriving on the sixth floor, we learned there were no beds available. Often, patients who were scheduled for discharge were unable to leave at the last minute.

Ross visited with friends who were back on the hall. The staff welcomed him with hugs and kisses. As we were leaving, we saw Kathy and Pat Holloway going toward the elevator.

"No bed for you either?" Ross asked.

"It's not that," Kathy replied. "My blood counts are too low for treatment. I'm going back home."

"Come home with us," Pat suggested. "We have no plans for the day."

"Let's do it, Mom," Ross said. "I don't want to go back to the hotel."

Pat arranged for Ross and Kathy to have lunch at a club. Since neither of them could eat, they opted for orange ices. We left them sitting under an umbrella by the pool, then we drove to Old Town Alexandria for lunch.

We strolled down the historic streets, browsed in the unique shops, and had lunch at a patio cafe. Both of us felt uneasy about leaving our grown-up children. Pat called her home to see if anyone had heard from Kathy and Ross, and learned that, not long after we had left, the hospital had called, frantically looking for Kathy. Further investigation of her blood work indicated her counts were critically low. Also, a bed had become available for Ross. Pat's son had driven to the club to get them and took them back to NIH. We wondered if we had experienced a lapse of sanity in trying to take a holiday.

In the late afternoon, efforts were begun to start Ross's prehydration. After the frustration and tension of finding a vein, the needle wouldn't stay in place. They gave up. Again, he was sent back to the hotel at 9:00 p.m. Tomorrow, the needle would have to be placed surgically in his neck vein. I knew Ross wouldn't sleep well that night.

∾

July, 1983

The next morning, as the surgical team laid out their instruments, Ross watched carefully, his body tense and his eyes worried. But soon the needle was firmly in place. Ross's tension and discomfort disappeared when he realized that his right hand was free.

The ability to use his hand, combined with the antiemetic drugs, helped him to fare much better with the next two rounds of treatment. In fact, he felt well enough to get out of bed afterward and walk around the hall, pushing the IV pole with his free right hand. He went up to the 14th floor recreation room with other patients and played pool. Between treatments, he visited Rock Creek Park, rode the metro to Capitol Hill, and even went to a rock concert with Kathy and her brother. He was a little woozy and weak, but his spirits were good.

When hospitalized one Saturday, he suggested we go to the 14th floor for the weekend movie. When we arrived in the playroom-turned-theater, there were patients and caregivers of all ages and from all over the hospital. We selected a seat which would accommodate the IV pole and which gave us a clear view of the screen among all the other IV poles.

The film was *An Officer and a Gentleman*. After a few minutes into the show, I recalled something I had heard about this story. Evidently, the movies shown on the 14th floor had not been checked for ratings. Ross laughed and teased me about my embarrassment during the torrid sexual scenes.

∾

It was the Fourth of July. Back in our hotel, we woke to thunder and lightning. In every direction, dark clouds swirled. We dashed out to the car and returned to NIH for blood work. Ross met his new Clinical Associate, again a female.

From the hospital, we drove to McLean, Virginia, where we

boarded the metro and rode to the Ballston station. After riding up the unusually long escalator, we stepped out into hard rainfall. Mary and Frank picked us up and drove to Capitol Hill where they managed to find a parking space.

Sound, mature thinking escaped me as we moved with mobs of people to the Capitol steps in the rain. Intermittently, the rain stopped, giving us hope that the weather would clear. Ross wore his hat and a jacket. In the mass of people, an umbrella proved to be a hindrance.

The fireworks, marvelously exciting when combined with streaks of lightning, created an awesome spectacle which eased my guilty conscience for allowing Ross to be exposed to the rain and the crowds. The rolling drums competed with the thunder as thousands of people sang *The Star Spangled Banner.*

The next day, Kathy drove her car to pick up Ross at the hotel and they went together to the Clinic for blood work. When finished, they went to the main street of Bethesda, where they strolled and window-shopped. Kathy wore a perky sun hat and a new blue sundress trimmed in white lace.

They were gone for three hours, and when Kathy returned Ross to the hotel, they sat by the pool under an umbrella with their heads close together, whispering and laughing.

Since Ross would be returning to Mobile for the next two rounds of treatment, this would be their farewell date. They promised to write and telephone each other.

16

The July heat bore down on Mobile when we arrived home. Ross was restless, cross, grumpy, and bored as he moped around the house. Most of his friends had summer jobs. He missed the constant telephone calls and visitors.

Then Don Mosley called to tell him that his parents had given him a graduation gift of a trip to the Virgin Islands. He asked Ross to go with him.

The next morning, Ross popped out of bed a little earlier than usual with a remarkable improvement in his mood.

I shook my head and said, "It's completely out of the question, Ross, and you know it. Don't even think of such a thing. Your white blood count is dropping now."

He picked up the phone and dialed. "This is Ross. Let me speak to Dr. Clarkson, please."

I stepped near the phone and leaned my head so I could eavesdrop. Ross turned his back to me, but I could still hear.

He told the doctor about the proposed trip and asked what he thought about the possibility.

"When did you want to go, Ross?"

"Saturday."

"Which Saturday?"

"This Saturday."

"Are you serious? That would be very risky, Ross. Are you sure you want to take this chance?"

"I really want to go, Dr. Clarkson. I'll take my chances."

After a brief period of silence, Dr. Clarkson said, "Go ahead, Ross, and have a good time. Take a thermometer and don't get sunburned."

Ross hung up the phone and turned to me. "I'm going, Mom. Okay? He said I could. I'll be careful. You don't have to worry."

The phone rang and I answered it.

"Mrs. Phelps? Dr. Clarkson. Tell Ross that he must wear shoes at all times, even in the water. He must not go barefoot. He must not eat any raw foods—none whatsoever—no fruits, salads—nothing. Everything has to be cooked."

"I'm very uneasy about this," I said.

"It's not the best time for him to be trying this, but if he's very careful, he'll be okay."

"What if he has a problem—a fever, or a cut or something?"

"Tell him not to see any doctor on the island—no matter what happens. Tell him to get to Miami the best way he can and call me. I'll locate someone down there for him to see."

Ross went to the bank, withdrew almost all of his graduation gift money, and he and Don left Mobile at 8:00 Saturday morning, driving to Atlanta in my car. There, they caught their flight to St. Thomas.

On Friday, Don's father called to say that he had a telephone call from St. Thomas and the boys were having a great time. They had met the captain of a cruise sailing ship who had offered them a job. Don wanted to stay and join the crew but wasn't sure if Ross should travel alone and make the drive from Atlanta to Mobile. I assured Dr. Mosley that Ross would make the right decision.

Ross reached Atlanta at 9:00 p.m. on Sunday, retrieved the car, and drove all the way to Mobile. He arrived home at 3:00 a.m., slept for a few hours, then got up early and went immediately to Dr. Clarkson's office for blood work. Afterward, he visited Don's parents to talk about the Virgin Islands. He took his film to a speedy developer and came home carrying his photos.

"Mom, come sit down. I want to show you the most beautiful place in the world. Look at that water! In some places, you could see fish—all kinds—seventy-five feet down. It was incredible."

They had rented a boat but didn't fish. They snorkeled, swam, and gazed at the underwater world.

"I covered myself with lotion and stayed inside during the middle of the day. Wait until you see Don. He looks like a native."

"A blond native? With blue eyes?"

"When he has dark glasses and a cap on. Mom, it was the prettiest place. You ought to go there. I wish the whole family could go. You would like it."

"Your dad isn't keen on sun and sand, fishing and boating."

He shrugged his shoulders. "He could sit in the shade and drink one of those tall fruit drinks with little paper umbrellas in them."

I looked at him from the corner of my eye. "And, what else? I believe there's something else in those drinks besides fruit juice and little umbrellas."

"They put rum in almost everything, I think. But the food was good. Before you ask, I didn't eat anything raw."

"How did you meet the captain of the boat?"

His face widened into a smile. "In a bar. He was real friendly and funny. He's all sunburned—traveled all over the world. His boat is huge and it's real nice, but the paint is peeling in a few places. Don is helping paint the hull. Then he's going to be a deckhand when they shove off in a couple of weeks."

"What kind of job did he offer you?"

He grinned and said, "Chef."

"Chef? I hardly think you're qualified for that."

"I'm just kidding. I told him I could cook—even with one hand. He said I could work in the galley."

"How long will Don stay gone?"

"As long as he wants to, I guess. This guy runs a charter for rich folks. They just take off and go and don't worry about anything." He turned and stared out the window. "I'm going back, Mom. Just as soon as I get over the treatment. I'm going to take off and not worry about anything."

ℳ

When he visited Dr. Clarkson for blood work, Ross learned that treatment could be given by Friday. On Thursday night, I found him in his room crying.

"I'm fed up with this, Mom," he said. "I want to get on with my life for whatever time I have left."

"I know...I know."

"If something else comes along, I want to do it. There's lots of things I want to do. I don't know if I'll have enough time. I don't want to pass up opportunities."

"I don't know what to tell you. I understand how you feel."

"No, you don't understand. Don't even say you do. You don't know what it's like to see all your friends doing the things you want to do."

"This will pass. If all goes well, you'll be through before you realize it."

"I'm not even near the end of treatment. Stop saying that! I can't take this anymore."

I sat on his bed and lifted his hand. He jerked it away.

"Just leave me alone!"

"Can you try to put all this out of your mind and get some sleep? We'll talk in the morning."

"Leave me alone. Get out of my room!"

I turned and walked away.

ℳ

Heavy sedation kept him in a semi-conscious state for this round of adriamycin and cis platin. I sat close by his bed near his head and watched for the quivering of his lips so I could know when to lift his head from the pillow and place the basin under his chin. I prayed that his sedation would prevent any knowledge or memory of the experience.

If at all possible, each time he was unhooked from the IV to get ready for discharge, I persuaded him to get out of bed and try to walk, hoping the exercise would help to clear his head of the antiemetic drugs. He placed his arm around my shoulder as we slowly walked along the hall until it was time to go. With each successive round of treatment, he leaned heavier and heavier on my shoulder.

∽

August, 1983

When Ross was discharged from the hospital and we reached our house, the phone was ringing. Pat Holloway was on the line. In a controlled voice, she told me that Kathy had suffered a seizure and was in a coma.

I handed the telephone to Ross and said, "It's Kathy's mom. Kathy is very sick."

He listened quietly as Pat gave him the details. He asked if it would help if he went to Bethesda to see Kathy. With understanding and compassion, Pat advised him not to come.

When he hung up the phone, he went to his room and closed the door. The next day, he sent Kathy a telegram, then mailed a special delivery letter.

Later in the week, I talked Scott into going with Ross and me to Gulf Shores for the annual gathering of the aunts and cousins. Scott felt he had outgrown this activity. He had been working too hard, and was having difficulty getting to sleep at night. It was as if he had a motor inside him which was set for full speed. Maybe, I thought, if he walked on the beach, looked at the horizon, and listened to the pounding surf, it would help to slow him down so he could relax.

Our group had rented two small houses side by side in order to keep the teenagers and little ones separated. My domain and responsibility was the teenage quarters. Our late nights were noisy, but, unlike the residents of the next-door cottage, we were able to sleep late.

Ross had to remain inside for most of the day, but after the sun went down, he was ready to join the on-going party. Scott actually enjoyed himself. He provided musical entertainment in the late evening by playing his guitar, and he even took responsibility for cooking for everybody one night—hamburgers on the grill.

When we arrived home from the beach, the phone was ringing. When I answered it, all I could hear was a weak, soft voice saying, "Ross." I handed him the phone to him and said, "I think it's Kathy."

He eagerly reached it, but after a few minutes, he slowly placed it back into its cradle and walked out the door, his eyes brimming. "I couldn't understand a word she said," he mumbled.

On August 23, the call came from Pat Holloway. Kathy had died that morning. She assured Ross that Kathy had received his letter. Pat had read it to her and Kathy had smiled when hearing his words.

A heavy, gray blanket of grief descended upon him and isolated him, and he couldn't discuss Kathy's death with me.

Each member of our family seemed to be isolated from the other. We had our own solitary sorrows, worries, and pain that we often coupled with demands on each other. Our whole family seemed to be falling apart, individually and as a unit. Mary came home to try to lend a hand.

She listened to me, and responded firmly and sometimes painfully. She tried to encourage her dad to express his feelings— we could see them in his tired, worried, and sad face and the far-away look in his eyes.

Our marriage had been on thin ice for more than a year before Ross's illness. Now, Bill and I had completely lost each other in the whirlwind surrounding us and our family. What little communication we once had now deteriorated into bickering and resentments. It seemed to me that he withdrew farther and farther from all of us, and I tried, unsuccessfully, to demand that he become involved, to be present. He criticized me for trying to do too much—for stretching myself too thin—which made me cross and irritable. He put up a thick wall around himself, and I bloodied my knuckles trying to break it down.

Into this chaos, Mary entered and tried to be the healer—the rescuer—of her family, a task that no one, probably not even a professional, could have accomplished.

She took Scott to New Orleans for a few days to give him a change of scene and offer support for the difficult time he was personally going through. Scott had always set high standards for himself, and worked like a slave to reach them. Then, when he failed to live up to his goals, he fell into despondency. He had been in a black hole for several weeks, and nothing I, or anyone else, said to him could relieve his anxieties. Reminders of his abilities, his good character, his talents, his friendships, and his extraordinary good looks were rejected.

Only his guitar offered solace. Both he and Ross had learned the guitar when they were young teenagers, and they often played together—usually some popular, loud rock number. Scott had excelled through many hours of practice, surpassing Ross in his ability. After Ross's amputation, Scott refused to even touch his guitar for several months, and when he finally picked it up again, he always went outside on the patio.

I could hear a different sound when he played—a soft strumming of a haunting, melancholy song. Here was a sadness and a wound that I couldn't soothe; a wall I didn't know how to break down; a darkness where I could shine no light.

When he and Mary returned from New Orleans, she drove Ross to the beach and brought him home in time to be admitted to the Mobile Infirmary for another round of adriamycin and cis platin. She and Scott visited Ross in the hospital, but they didn't stay long. It was their first time to observe Ross when getting a chemotherapy treatment. Before Mary left, she and Scott spent time at the beach.

Both Scott and Ross clung to her when they said good-bye at the Mobile airport. She kissed her dad and me. With a heavy heart, she boarded the plane to return to Washington to face her own personal challenges alone.

℘

September, 1983

Jim Phillips moved out of his mother's home and into an apartment. Ross had been trying to figure out a way to move away from home, and Jim had said they could share a place. Ross gathered boxes, placed them in the hall, and started collecting things from around the house.

Following his next round of chemotherapy treatment, he started packing and loading the car. On the big day, I helped him haul loads of things the short distance away. He planned to cook all his meals at the apartment, so we made a big trip to the grocery. The complex didn't allow animals, so I promised I would be responsible for Rocky.

Ross stopped by the house often to do his laundry, check his mail, and play with Rocky. One day, when he came into the house, he said, "Mom, what do you think about you and me driving over to New Orleans and spending the night with Aunt Dorothy?"

"Fine, I guess. What brought this on?"

"I've been invited to a big party over at Tulane. I'd like to go, but I don't feel like riding with anybody or partying all night. We could drive over, I could go to the party for awhile, and then spend the night with Aunt Dorothy."

"Sounds reasonable to me. I'd enjoy it. Dorothy and I love to go into the Quarter and have gumbo at one of those little cafes. Let's call her."

As he drove along Interstate 10, I asked, "How's apartment life? Everything going okay?"

"Yes. I like it. But I'm not getting any rest. There's always a gang over there. I'm so tired."

"Maybe it'll settle down."

"I doubt it. All our friends who still live at home like to hang out over there and party all night."

"You can sleep at home if you need to."

"I'm not moving home."

"I didn't say that. You could come home when you get tired and sleepy and then go back in the morning."

"There's nothing to do in the daytime. Jim goes to work. If I came home to sleep, somebody else would sleep in my bed. I don't like that."

He agreed to change the radio dial to music that I enjoyed and we rode quietly for a few miles.

"Mom, do you know what type cancer Mike Murawa had?"

"No. If it was ever known, his mother didn't tell me. You know he was sick for over a year before he came to NIH."

"Why? Why didn't they start treatment earlier?"

"I don't think they knew it was cancer. He had been in treatment for something else, I think. I really don't know."

"What about Kathy? Do you know anything about her disease?"

"Very little. I don't remember her mom saying the exact name of the tumor. All I know is that it was in her brain, and, as far as I know, she didn't have surgery."

"Why not? There's hardly any place in the brain where they can't do surgery."

"I don't know, Ross. Maybe it had spread. I don't know."

"She had lots of radiation and chemotherapy."

"You can't compare yourself to either Mike or Kathy. Every case is different. You had an early diagnosis. Your surgery most definitely removed the tumor, and you started treatment immediately. Every case is different...."

"Looks like they all end the same way."

"That's not true."

"They both had chemotherapy, and they had radiation which I've never had."

"I don't think either of them had surgery. I don't understand anything about it. The doctors can't answer those questions. There's no point in trying to figure it out."

We dropped that subject and quietly listened to music on the radio. It was a beautiful, late summer day.

As we were nearing the Louisiana state line, he suddenly said, "Mom, I've been meaning to tell you. I don't want to die in a hospital, and I don't want to be buried in a cemetery."

I sighed, looked out the window, and wondered how I could get him off this subject. But, maybe it was best for him to verbalize his thoughts. "I don't either, Ross. Please keep that in mind when I die. But I think there are laws about where people can be buried. Also, please see to it that no unnecessary money is spent on my burial. I want a simple pine box."

We rode silently for the rest of the way to New Orleans, and he attended the party at Tulane while I visited with Dorothy. When we returned to Mobile the next evening, he played with Rocky for awhile, then went to the apartment.

Later that week, Pat Holloway sent me a copy of the letter Ross had written to Kathy before she died. She felt I should know the depth of Ross's thoughts and feelings.

It was dated August 7, 1983:

> "...I don't really know what to say to you except that I care a lot about you. You mean very much to me. I want to tell you about the way I pray to God about you and myself. I have often heard people say that a positive attitude can beat cancer. When I was down awhile back, I would picture a bright light in my mind. It's the healing power of God to me. I would picture this light in my mind and imagine it flowing into me and try my hardest to feel it throughout me. This is something that I seem to be able to do with ease now and I wanted to share it with you. Try this if you wish, and try to feel the contentment and comfort I have felt. Your faith is so important! This method is all I use for myself because I know of nothing else stronger or anything else I can do, personally, to help myself. I put all of my faith and hope into it for you.
>
> "I say you are special to me because I've never met a girl like you before. You see things my way, and I in turn think I know what you're about. Between what you and I have been through, I think we both understand each other very well.
>
> "...Please remember that I pray for you every day.

Please also let me know if there is anything, anything at all I can do for you, ANYTHING!

"...Please get in touch with me soon. I miss you. My mom sends her love and prayers. You're in my thoughts, Sunshine. All of my love to you, Ross."

17

School had begun at UMS Prep and the yearbooks from the previous year were in the office. Ross went to school to get his copy and came home, sat on the patio, and pored over it for a long time. In addition to the usual pictures and snapshots, the seniors had dedicated a page to Ross with an inspiring message, along with photos of him from the earlier grades through high school. He wasn't expecting this.

On September 18, his 19th birthday, we went to church. Afterward, he, his date, and the whole family went to the Grand Hotel at Point Clear for lunch. When we returned home, he announced that he and Rocky were going to the park because he had to do some serious thinking. No one questioned him.

Monday morning, he walked into the kitchen and asked me to sit down. "I've decided to stop treatment," he said, watching my face closely. "I've been thinking about it a lot."

"I know you have."

"I want to know what you think of it. Do you think it's all right?"

"I sure don't know what's right. But it's okay with me. I don't blame you at all."

"I've had about forty treatments."

"Thirty-nine to be exact."

"And I have four more. But I can't take it anymore. I want to stop."

"That suits me," I told him. "Let's go see Dr. Clarkson."

Dr. Clarkson did not seem to be surprised. He didn't disagree, explaining that the best results from chemo were the first dosages, the up-front treatments. The risks involved with future treatments could very well be greater than any good they might do. He suggested we return to NIH to discuss the matter.

Ross was only slightly relieved, and he became very frightened. He took the *Physician's Desk Reference* from the bookshelf and again read all the damage his drugs could cause. Maybe the problems he had would be reversible if treatment stopped now. He talked and pondered. He paced and fidgeted. He went outside and played with Rocky, then came in the house with tear-stained eyes.

"Why don't you wait until you talk to the doctors at NIH and see what their reaction is?" Bill asked.

"They'll try to make me continue," Ross stated.

"You're the one to make the decision, no matter what they say, but let's hear them out," I said. "They can't make you continue. It's your life."

He asked permission from our friends, Don and Nonnie Muller, to use their beach house, and left that afternoon to spend the night. At some point that evening, he made his decision. He was through. He would take no more.

After midnight, he decided to drive back home. After reloading his car, he discovered he had locked his car keys inside the beach house.

Even under normal circumstances, Ross often showed little patience. I could picture his anger—his lips pulled tight, breathing in short breaths, pacing, balling up his fist.

I could imagine his explosion as he slammed his right hand through a glass pane near the door knob. He cut the artery in his wrist.

Frantically, he called Dr. Clarkson at home. Dr. Clarkson told him that somehow, he would have to figure out a way to put pressure over the artery to stop the bleeding. He told him to call home.

At 3:00 a.m. he called and I heard Bill talking to him. "Come on home, Ross. There's nothing we can do from over here. Calm down. Just come on home and I'll go over tomorrow to fix the glass in the door."

"What's happened? What's the matter?" I asked.

"He's cut his wrist real bad."

"Cut his wrist? Let me talk to him!"

Bill handed me the phone.

"Ross, what's wrong?"

"My wrist...I cut my wrist real bad...blood is shooting out of it...."

"What happened? Never mind. Do you have your prosthesis on?"

"Yes, I'm trying to put pressure on it but it's still bleeding real bad. I don't know if I can drive."

"Just try to stop the bleeding. I'm on my way. Don't try to drive...stay right there."

Hanging up the phone, I said to Bill, "Come on, let's hurry!"

"Just calm down. It's not necessary to go charging over to the Gulf at three o'clock in the morning."

"We've got to do something! Maybe we should send an ambulance. Hurry, let's go!"

We threw on clothes, raced to the car, and headed for the interstate. When we left the main highway on the farm-to-market roads, Bill faithfully obeyed the speed limits. There was no traffic anywhere.

"Will you please drive faster? Just once in your life, break the law—exceed the speed limit!"

"Why don't you calm down? Why in the world did he do that?"

"He's terribly upset, Bill. He's scared, angry, confused."

"You shouldn't have let him go over there by himself if he's that upset. Why didn't he use his prosthesis to break the window, or a piece of wood or something."

I wanted to scream at him. "He's upset, Bill."

Through thick branches of pine trees, I could see lights in the cottage when we turned down the palmetto lined, sandy road. We opened the door and saw Ross lying on the sofa with his eyes closed. There was blood everywhere—on his face, his clothes, the walls, floors, and kitchen counter.

Bill reached down and touched Ross. He gasped a deep breath and started crying. "He's dead."

I bent down to kiss Ross's face and felt his breath against my cheek. "He's not dead! Call an ambulance! Call the police! Call anybody!"

While Bill reached for the phone, I grabbed a bathcloth, wet it, and patted Ross's face. He remained totally still.

"Ross...Ross," I whispered. "Dad and I are here. You're going to be okay."

Bill paced back and forth.

"Go out and watch for the ambulance. They might not see the road," I said.

"Can you take his pulse?" he asked.

"I don't know anything about that. I don't know how to find a pulse anywhere except in a wrist."

Bill pressed his fingers on the artery in Ross's neck. "I feel something. It feels like a pulse," he said.

The police arrived, and when they looked at the scene, they quickly moved into position to block the doors, expecting someone to try to make a fast get-away. I think they planned to handcuff Bill and me.

"What's happened here? Is this your place?"

"We're not real sure what happened. We just got here from Mobile," Bill said. "This is our son. He called to tell us he had an accident."

"The ambulance from Foley is on the way," an officer said. "I need a statement."

"I can tell you what he told us when he called," Bill said. "That's all we know. See—here's where he broke the glass with his fist. He cut the artery."

I had washed the blood off Ross's face and he began to rouse a bit. He whimpered as he lay there—eyes opening slightly, then closing again. When the siren blared down the driveway, he opened his eyes and asked, "What's that?"

"It's the ambulance—we're going to get you to a hospital. You're going to be okay."

"Oh, Mom...I'm sorry to cause so much trouble. An ambulance isn't necessary. I can ride in a car."

"Just be very still. Don't move. The bleeding may start again."

Bill and I followed the flashing light to the Foley hospital where a compassionate doctor stitched Ross's wrist. The man showed patience and understanding. Later, he came out into the hall and told me that his little girl had recently died of neuroblastoma, a form of cancer.

We drove 10 miles back to the beach to get Ross's things and the other car. Ross rode home with me, crying most of the way. His decision had been reached. He was finished, but he was terrified.

The next morning, he called Dr. Poplack and told him of his decision. Dr. Poplack told him to come up for conferences.

In our limited understanding of cancer treatment, for all we knew, stopping the drugs could open the door for the return of the disease. On the other hand, he may never have had any errant cells, and the treatment may not have been necessary to start with.

Ross's athletic physique had deteriorated to a mere skeleton covered with white skin. One day, as I watched him in the yard playing with Rocky, I thought he looked like a skinny little bird with no feathers—and missing part of its wing.

On Saturday, Mary met Ross at Dulles and tried to keep him calm. Bill and I returned to the Muller's beach house with scrub brushes and sponges and spent the day cleaning the cottage. Bill replaced the broken glass and we returned home.

On Sunday, I flew to Maryland and the next day, Ross and I met with five different doctors. Ross asked each of them the same questions over and over. "How important is it to take the last four treatments? What would happen if I had a metastasis? What are my chances now? Do you think it's okay if I stop?"

No one could give a definite answer to any of his questions, but no one discouraged him from quitting. He cried off and on all day. It seemed he couldn't stop.

As many times as I had been there, I had never formally met the Chief Pediatric Oncologist, Dr. Philip Pizzo. I had seen him with the groups making rounds. From what I understood, if anyone had a problem with any member of the staff, he or she could take it up with Dr. Pizzo. Since Ross would have forbidden me to do such a thing, I had never asked to see him. This time, without checking with Ross, I asked for an appointment. Ross went with me to his office.

"Obviously," he said, "I believe in chemotherapy. We know it can often produce a remission. However, history will look back on this era as being barbaric. Unfortunately, at this time, we have nothing else."

"What do you think about my stopping now, with four more treatments to go?" Ross asked. "Dr. Clarkson thinks it's okay."

"I agree with Dr. Clarkson, Ross. It's the early diagnosis and the quick treatment that produces good results. I have no problem whatsoever with your stopping the treatment now."

"Dr. Pizzo, what you think causes cancer," I asked.

"I think it's environmental," he said. "And that includes the air we breathe, the food we eat, the water we drink, the clothes we wear, and every other aspect of our lives."

As we left his office with his endorsement to stop the treatment, I wondered what in the environment could be worse than the chemicals that had been pumped into Ross's body. But I was relieved that not one single person had told him he should continue. His part of the study would not be affected.

Since there were so few patients in the study, I thought about the other participants and whether any other patient had actually completed the protocol, but I didn't ask. I wondered how many had died of the disease or from the treatment. Although the question was never raised, I learned later that all new patients were put on the same protocol that Ross had, with some desperately needed modifications.

That afternoon, I returned home, leaving Ross with Mary. He planned to return to NIH for blood work and urinalyses in an effort to find a way to control the magnesium depletion. Between trips to NIH, he went to work with Mary and wandered around the District. He composed a song as a tribute to Kathy.

Over a year had passed since diagnosis. When Ross returned home on Sunday, he seemed a little calmer and didn't want to discuss it anymore.

∾

October, November, December, 1983

After Ross returned to Mobile, he began to spend more and more time at home instead of at the apartment. He was lonely and his moods fluctuated. Jim wasn't home much because of his college study and a part-time job, and I knew that he caught the brunt of a lot of Ross's frustrations.

One Sunday afternoon while we sat on the patio, I asked, "Is something wrong? You look kind of down."

He reached down and picked up an acorn and tossed it across the patio. "I'm going through a bad time, Mom. I don't want to talk about it."

"How can I help you if you don't want to tell me? You and Jim getting along okay?"

"No, we're not. But I don't want to talk about it."

"Okay. I'm not interested in the details."

"You don't understand, Mom. Nobody understands."

"Understands what?"

"What I've been through...everything."

"There's no way anybody could understand. I was with you more than anyone and even I don't understand. You can't expect your friends to understand."

He rose and slowly paced around the patio table. "I can't do a lot of things, Mom...at least, not easily. It's hard for me to do a lot of things."

"Like what? I think you do very well."

"I don't want to have to ask Jim to do things for me. But I can't carry bulky things that take two hands. It takes me longer to bathe and get dressed."

"Is that a problem for Jim? Has he said anything about it?"

"No, he hasn't said anything, but I can tell. He's always in a big hurry. I don't want to talk about it."

"You'll feel better, Ross. As you said, this is only a bad time you're going through—temporary."

"I don't want to have to live with you and Dad all my life. I want to live on my own like everybody else."

"So do we, Ross. So do we. We're not planning on you getting stuck at home. You're managing fine. Quit worrying about it."

He sat back down, propped his elbow on his knee, and covered his eyes with his hand. "Maybe I should look for my own place so I won't be such a big bother to Jim."

"Give this arrangement with Jim a chance, Ross. Do your part to keep the peace. Jim has been the best friend a guy could have. He's understanding, loyal and true..."

"Sometimes he doesn't understand."

"He has feelings, too, Ross. Ever think about that? You've been so busy with your own problems that maybe you should take a look at Jim and see what his problems are."

"I do, Mom. How do you think we became good friends? We always talk about our problems with each other."

He bent his head down and rubbed his forehead, shielding his eyes. Then he got up and walked around the patio and said, "I think I'll sleep at home tonight."

"Okay. But tomorrow..."

"Let me handle my own affairs, Mom."

He slept at home most of the time with occasional visits to the apartment to get something he needed. But by December, he began to feel much better. He and Jim cleared the air with their differences and he spent more time in the evenings at their apartment. Friends invited him on weekend trips to their colleges. His time at home was only to eat, do laundry, play with Rocky, or sit at the piano picking out a tune.

Thanksgiving came and went; Christmastime was near. We decorated the tree on Scott's birthday; Mary arrived home. Ross shopped with Mary and she helped him get Rocky to the vet for sprucing up for the holidays.

On Christmas Eve, I dashed out to the mall for some final shopping. As I was hurrying toward the exit, I saw a lady pushing a girl in a wheelchair. I walked several steps before it registered with me that the girl had only one arm and that the lady looked familiar. Slowing my pace, I turned, retraced my steps and said, "Excuse me...."

"Elaine," the lady said. "How are you?"

"Ann? Ann Dungan?" I said. "I was walking so fast, and I don't have my glasses on...I didn't recognize you. Lana, it's good to see both of you."

Ann stood straight, looked firmly at me and smiled. "We're doing some of Lana's last-minute shopping."

I didn't ask how Lana was feeling or what was going on with her. I didn't have to. She only faintly resembled the vivacious teenager who had visited Ross a little more than a year before.

Ann's sad eyes were not hidden by her fixed smile. She said, "We're pretty worn out from all the Christmas shopping and are on our way to the car. I hope everything is all right with Ross."

"He's okay—finished treatment in August and hopes to start college soon."

"Have a good Christmas," Lana said. "Tell Ross I said hello."

"I will, Lana. Come to see us."

I turned and walked in the other direction.

When I reached home, the Riordas had arrived from New Orleans to spend the night. Ross decided to sleep at home on a pallet in front of the fire. It was a reminder of previous Christmas Eves when there were wall-to-wall people on beds, sofas and sleeping bags in our home.

In earlier years, when our children were small, Dorothy's husband, Joe Riorda, and Bill began a tradition of taking all the little ones to an early afternoon movie on Christmas Eve.

Dorothy and I stayed in the kitchen preparing the holiday meals. The children and their daddies usually saw a James Bond thriller, and although I questioned the suitability of these films for small children, they had a marvelous time and teased me for being a fuddy-duddy. When they returned home, full of laughter and chatter about the movie, Dorothy and I dressed them in their best clothes and took them to a mall for a picture of the six of them with Santa Claus. By that time of day, very few shoppers were about, and the stores were being prepared for closing.

During the annual excursion when Ross was three years old, we had finished the picture-taking and were wandering through the mall, letting the children romp off their energy. One by one, the stores became darkened as they closed.

We rounded up the children in preparation to leave. When we counted heads, someone was missing—Ross. We couldn't spot him in the almost empty mall. I found a security guard and he joined in the search. Dorothy and I, with children in tow, separated and began to look in the stores that remained open. The other kids made a game of it, running around calling, "Ross...Ross... Where are you? Santa's coming...."

In the distance, I spotted a store which still had a light on, and I ran toward it. The bookstore cashier reminded me that the store was closed.

Rushing around the aisles, I found Ross, completely hidden in a corner behind a large box of rolls of Christmas wrapping paper, sitting on the floor, lost in a book.

With relief and irritation, I said, "Ross, we're leaving! Why didn't you stay with us? Everybody's been looking for you! We were scared...we'd lost you."

I had interrupted his concentration on his book and he slowly turned his head and calmly looked up at me with complete trust. "You didn't lose me, Mama. I'm not lost. I'm in Bookland. I knew you wouldn't leave me."

PART TWO

January, 1984—May, 1988

18

By January, 1984, Ross felt stronger and looked much better. He had gained weight and had a little color in his cheeks. His hair began to slowly come back but we weren't certain exactly what color it would be, or if it would be straight or curly. It appeared very dark, almost black, which didn't fit my memory of how he once looked. As his hair grew, it looked shaggy and unkempt, so he agreed to go with me to my hairdresser, Margaret Botter, for advice. The new growth appeared in spots with questionable direction, and the color was a mixture of black and brown. Tight curls emerged in scattered spots. Margaret took on the challenge of trying to keep him satisfied.

He registered at Spring Hill College, and, when classes began, he popped into the house often. He was enthusiastic about his courses and all the people he met. He signed up for a full load with special tutoring in some classes, started voice lessons, and joined the chorale. A music teacher patiently helped him with piano, and he spent hours singing to the top of his lungs. In the evenings, he took Rocky to obedience school and started an exercise regimen for himself.

We had been told that it could take a full year to recuperate from chemotherapy, but after only four months, he had progressed very well. He had limited stamina, which disappointed him, but he tried to keep up with his friends. He didn't have to return to NIH until the end of March, and would get an X-ray of his chest at the Mobile Infirmary once a month. The magnesium depletion finally cleared several months later, the cramps lessened, and he stopped taking the handful of tablets except when needed.

Since Ross had moved into the apartment and signed up for his heavy college schedule, it had been difficult for me to gear down to a normal life. I wasn't even certain what "normal" would be anymore. Bill and I made an effort to agree to a tentative truce, but there remained long periods of silence. Although we stayed together, we were alone and unable, or unwilling, to communicate our fears and pain with each other.

Scott had moved back home a few months after Ross had moved out, so my household responsibilities remained the same—the shopping, cooking, laundry, and housekeeping chores. But, for a large part of the day, I was alone, and it seemed strange.

The stack of inspirational and psychological self-help books which had been handed to me remained on the shelf, but a small, thin paperback I had owned for many years proved to be the most important book in my possession. *The Will of God,* by Leslie Weatherhead, differentiated in clear language his understanding of God's intentional will, His circumstantial will, and His ultimate will. With the help of God, Ross and the rest of us were living in His circumstantial will.

Around the middle of February, a job offer came to me to work in a political campaign for a man running for congress. The fast-paced, stressful position with big responsibilities kept my mind occupied. I didn't have time to worry.

Ross made good friends on campus, and often went on weekend retreats conducted by priests and student leaders. He'd had Catholic friends in the past, and now he got a closer look at some of their beliefs.

He took a more serious interest in music. Although he had been exposed to the classics and could tolerate them to a point, he began to appreciate them as he learned more about theory. *Canon in D* by Johann Pachelbel became a favorite, and he bought several tapes with different instrumental combinations of the haunting, beautiful sounds.

He had made plans to be away from Mobile during the coming summer, and since I was working such long hours, he was concerned about Rocky. He started a rigorous training of the dog. Rocky was leash trained, but we didn't know what he would do if ever he got out of our fenced-in yard. Ross took him out with the leash daily, often letting him loose, and tried to teach him to "heel." Rocky was a happy, joyful, jumping dog, and appeared to be skipping down the street with a big smile on his face.

One day, while I was getting a haircut from Margaret, Ross walked into the salon. "Rocky's dead," he said.

They had been on their usual training walk. When Ross unhooked the leash, Rocky spotted some other dogs and immediately romped off to play. The pack turned a corner and were out of sight. Ross knew Rocky could find his way home, so he went there to wait for him.

While in the front yard watching for him, our postman drove up into our driveway. He got out of his truck and told Ross he had just seen Rocky get hit by a car on Old Shell Road. He drove Ross in the mail truck back to Old Shell.

While Ross was standing in the street as his beloved friend lay still on the pavement, a kind lady drove by and saw what had happened. She assisted in putting the big animal in the trunk of her car and they drove to the veterinarian's clinic. It was too late. There wasn't a mark on him, but death had been instantaneous.

Ross called a friend to assist in getting Rocky from the veterinary hospital. Other friends came to the house to help. Using only his right arm, Ross labored with the shovel, sweat and tears streaming down his face, while he dug a proper grave in the back yard. Later, he planted a memorial tree over Rocky's grave.

∾

Before the end of the 1984 spring quarter, Ross had applied for an internship with our representative in Washington and was accepted into the program. The congressman had announced his intention to retire at the end of the year, and the man I worked for was running for that seat. Before Ross left for Washington, he moved all his things from the apartment back into the house.

He shopped for two new suits and a sport coat. In addition to the Capitol Hill experience as an intern, he had the good fortune to be able to stay in the home of the congressman's administrative assistant in Washington. Ross house-sat often for him, taking care of his dog and his big sedan, sometimes chauffeuring the congressman's wife to appointments.

While serving this internship, he saw a man he had met the summer he was in Washington taking care of Mary. He offered Ross another internship, this time with a senator from North Carolina. Ross came home at the end of the summer, again reluctantly, and wistfully said that he wished he could go to college in Washington and work on Capitol Hill.

During the time he was gone, he called home weekly, full of chatter about his activities. I had not told him that Lana Dungan had died in July. After he arrived home, I broke the news to him and I also told him of an incredible phenomenon which had occurred in the Dungan family. Karen Dungan, Lana's older sister, had just been diagnosed with osteosarcoma in the same place as Lana—the shoulder.

"That can't be true. It's not possible," he said.

"That's what I was told by your Aunt Jean."

"Has Karen had surgery or is she in treatment?"

"I understand she decided not to have an amputation but she's getting chemotherapy."

"Oschner's?" he asked.

"I don't know. Lana switched to M. D. Anderson in Texas several months before she died."

"I didn't know that. I can't believe the same thing has

happened to her sister. That's bizarre...," he said, slowly shaking his head. "Are you sure, Mom?"

"Ask Aunt Jean. Ask Dr. Clarkson. I'm sure he's heard about it."

"I'll talk to Aunt Jean...," he said, as he turned and walked away.

∽

In the fall of 1984, Ross began his college studies in earnest, admitting that, for the first time in his life, he had learned how to study. He spent all his evenings in the library.

With Ross living at home again, Scott had decided to move out into an apartment again. He had a job and was taking classes at night. I recalled the remark of my witty friend, Hazel Mayson, when her children were this age that they "wore out the doors moving in and out."

Family members met when passing through the house. We rarely sat together and talked until Sunday lunch, when we caught up with each other's activities. I now had something to report, since I had a job on the staff of the newly-elected congressman from the First District of Alabama. When H. L. "Sonny" Callahan was elected in November to the U. S. House of Representatives, I helped establish his district office in Mobile.

Ross's check-ups at NIH continued, but there was more time between tests. For the following year, 1985, he was scheduled for only two returns to NIH for X-rays and scans. It had been more than two years since diagnosis.

He was invited to go home with friends throughout the country, and he traveled in January to San Diego with Ann Smith, a Spring Hill coed, to visit her friends. A few days before they left on their trip, Ross's cat, Maggie, gave birth to five kittens.

Maggie had been given to Ross by one of his professors. She had been a part of a litter that was left orphaned when the mother was killed by a car.

Maggie and I met one evening when I returned home from

work. Ross sat in the living room, very still, wearing a jacket zipped almost to the top under his chin.

"What are you doing in here? Why do you have your jacket on?"

"Nothing, just sitting here," he said with a grin.

"Come on, Ross. What do you have under that jacket?"

He slowly unzipped it, and I saw what I thought was a tiny mouse, snuggled under his arm.

"Relax, Mom. It's just a baby kitten. I'll take care of it. You won't have to do a thing."

"Hah! That'll be the day. I'm not having any part of this, Ross. You're not a little kid. You're twenty years old. You know better. I don't have time for this and you don't either."

But he rushed home between classes each day to lift Maggie from the shoebox and feed her with an eyedropper. As she grew older, she became playful and tried to be friends with Mitty, the cat Mary had pawned off on us when she moved to Washington. But Mitty didn't like the intrusion into her space and hissed her disapproval.

As time went by, Ross promised that everything would be taken care of—not to worry. He did get some of the basics done, and saw to it that Maggie got her shots. He kept fresh flea collars on her. He got too busy, however, to have her fixed.

Soon, she was obviously pregnant and Ross became as excited as a little child. Finally, a few days before he and Ann were to leave for San Diego, Maggie appeared, slimmed down considerably.

Ross searched everywhere for the babies. He tried to follow Maggie to no avail. The weather had turned freezing cold and he worried that her kittens would die from starvation or freezing. Maggie was hardly more than a kitten herself, and Ross wasn't sure she would be responsible.

The day before he and Ann left on their trip, he heard the kittens mewing. They were inside the wall of a bedroom. Somehow, Maggie had gotten into the crawl space under the eaves and deposited her babies there. There was no way to get them out of the wall short of cutting a hole in the eave.

Ross felt better about Maggie's mothering ability and left on his trip. He called home twice to find out if Maggie had brought them out. She had not.

The night he and Ann arrived back in Mobile, Bill and I had guests. We were sitting in the living room when they walked in, happy to be back and full of information about all the things they had done and seen.

Ross sat down on the sofa and asked about Maggie. I opened the door and called her, leaving the door opened a bit.

Soon Maggie came in and deposited a baby kitten at Ross's feet. She looked up at him and mewed as he patted her on the head and spoke softly to her. She hastily retreated back out the door and returned with another. Then another, and another. When she came in with the fifth one, I closed the door.

The little blind babies moved shakily all over the living room floor between our guests' feet, but Maggie climbed into Ross's lap. Now we had seven cats.

Ross became the overseer of the kittens, rushing in between classes to be sure everyone was being taken care of. Soon they were weaned, and he found a home for two of them on campus. This left three babies, plus Maggie and Mitty. One poor baby met it's fate under the wheel of a car in our driveway, but the other two established their residence in our home.

19

In the summer of 1985, when Ross was planning his trip to NIH for his six-month check-up, he remembered having heard about a camp for children with cancer in Front Royal, Virginia. Patients who were able to travel to the camp were taken on day trips from NIH. He decided he would like to be a camp counselor.

He called Andy Tartler at NIH, and Andy promised he would check into it. Later, Andy called back and said, "Sorry, Ross. You need to have experience as a camper before they'll take you as a counselor."

Ross was very disappointed. Nurses and doctors from NIH helped staff Camp Fantastic and he felt certain there must be something he could do. He had an ability to relate to the young patients on the hall and thought he could be useful.

Later, Andy called back and said, "Ross, I've checked again, and they said they would love to have you as a camper. Why don't you plan to come on up?"

"Who ever heard of a twenty-year-old first-time camper, Andy? I can't do that."

However, he packed a few camp clothes when he left for NIH. Later in the week, he called to say his tests were all clear, and he didn't have to return for a whole year. Again, he was told that, if a metastasis is going to occur, it most often will happen within two years of onset. It had been almost three years.

From NIH he went to Camp Fantastic and returned to Mobile

two weeks later. He was jubilant about the experience. Although he couldn't adequately verbalize his feelings about the camp, I could tell that something very special must have happened there. Each time he discussed Camp Fantastic, his eyes lit up.

"You can go again next year as a counselor instead of a camper," I said.

"No way. It's much more fun to be a camper!"

Camp Fantastic emphasized a program of exercise, and Ross vigorously continued the plan which had been designed especially for him. He started doing push-ups on the floor, and though his left arm was weak, he persisted in trying to build it up. Not long after getting into this routine, the stump end of the left arm started hurting badly. We made an appointment with Dr. Pat Daugherty who, along with his partner Dr. King, had discovered the tumor in Ross's wrist in 1982.

Because of doing push-ups with the stump of his arm, a spur had formed on the end of the bone and was about to break through the skin. The bone wasn't strong enough for this activity. Dr. Daugherty scheduled surgery in an out-patient clinic and recommended there be no further such exercises.

The spur was clipped off and Ross's arm re-stitched while he was under heavy sedation. A pretty young nurse stood by him during the short procedure, holding his hand and listening while he groggily rambled on about college, girl friends, and his future plans.

After the surgery was finished and his head began to clear from the sedation, his nurse called me into the surgery room and handed me an emesis basin. She said, "Ross, you'll probably feel nauseated in a few minutes but don't worry about it. You're mom is here to help you, so you be very still for a few more minutes."

"You don't have to worry about me throwing up," he said through a sleepy haze. "That's one thing I know how to do."

He babbled on about a girl, telling me much more than he would have had he been fully awake. He had met her while on a retreat and fallen in love.

When I met Sandra later, it was obvious that she cared deeply for Ross. A pretty, soft-voiced girl, her deep-set green eyes gazed at him as she clasped his hand whenever they walked together.

They laughed softly while whispering secret messages. Although about the same age as Ross, Sandra seemed much younger, and Ross took a protective role when with her. She also sang in the chorale, so they were together at practice, at Sunday morning mass in St. Joseph's Chapel, and every other moment they could find.

He didn't notice that three years had passed since diagnosis.

ॐ

At the beginning of the 1986 winter quarter at Spring Hill, Ross became Resident Associate, which meant that he could live in the dorm without paying the expensive fees.

We shopped for things to furnish his large room in Murray Hall. He had to be available for other students and wanted his room to look comfortable and inviting. We visited yard sales and found two big stuffed chairs and a remnant of bright blue carpet. With his huge plants and a big jar of hard candy by the entrance, he opened his room for visiting students.

He enthusiastically entered activities and participated in several clubs. His friendships solidified and his grades improved. He worked hard and played hard—always in a hurry.

Because of his tight schedule, we rarely saw him, but I had no problem finding his laundry basket piled high and often found a few dirty dishes in the sink.

He joined us for the Easter family gathering at the Persons' farm—this year, a very painful reunion. James R. "Bud" Persons had been killed in the crash of a private plane the previous November while on a pheasant hunting trip to Kansas. Jean bravely carried on the tradition of the reunion, her two young sons standing beside her.

When the spring quarter ended, Ross continued summer school and also worked as counselor in the first camp for children with cancer in Mobile. Camp Rap-A-Hope, established by the Mobile County Medical Auxiliary, had 15 campers from South Alabama, South Mississippi and Northwest Florida. Ross was proud to be a part of the first Camp Rap-A-Hope.

20

When Ross's 1986 fall classes began, he often got behind on writing papers. He asked me to come to the computer lab at night to help him get caught up. Although he had learned the basics of using the computer with one hand, he was slow. He sat beside me and instructed me, point by point, on the use of the computer.

"Don't leave, Ross. I don't know what I'm doing on this thing."

"I'm not leaving. I'll be back in a minute. Just keep on doing what I told you."

"You write too small. I can't figure out some of the words. You've got to stay close by if you want my help."

"I'm only going to get a drink, Mom. I missed supper and I'm hungry."

"I missed supper, too. Let's take a break and get something to eat. This is going to take hours."

"Okay, but I don't want to go home. You'll get started doing something else and won't come back. I've got to turn this in tomorrow."

"You may have to pay somebody to do this computer work, Ross. I don't know what I'm doing and it makes me nervous."

"Relax, Mom. You're doing fine. Let's take a break and go to Hello Deli."

From this, we established a habit of going out to dinner every

Wednesday or Thursday—my nights to help him in the computer lab. Sitting in the little cafes nearby, he talked almost nonstop. There was so much on his mind that he never mentioned illness or difficulties with his amputation. Perhaps, since more than four years had passed, both he and I were beginning to let the nightmare recede into the past.

I dreaded bringing the subject up, but knew he would want to know that Karen Dungan had died. He said nothing when I told him, but later, he asked, "Karen Dungan did have surgery, didn't she?"

"Limb-sparing last year in January."

"Have you seen her mother?"

"No, your Aunt Jean keeps me informed."

"Do you know if anyone is going to research this—try to find out what happened?"

"I don't know. The Dungans aren't ready to talk about it."

"I'm not ready to talk about it, either."

When Ross was in a talking mood, he often spoke at length about things I knew nothing about. He was interested in China and the cultural revolution that had taken place there. He talked about the international monetary crisis, and the huge debts owed by Third World countries to banks in the United States.

He trusted me to proofread his papers and he marked clippings for me to cut from *The Wall Street Journal,* the *Christian Science Monitor* and several *Foreign Affairs* journals. While I learned a lot about world affairs, I also learned how difficult it is to cut clippings when using only one hand.

His focus solidified in the field of foreign relations. He joined the International Club on campus, where he got to know many foreign students. Since our house is near the campus, he planned gatherings of the International Club on our patio.

Several friends arrived at our house one Saturday morning to help plan and prepare food for a party. Shish-ka-bob was a favorite, and they sat around the kitchen table threading the sticks, making hundreds of small ka-bobs for grilling.

The kitchen was overcrowded, so I went upstairs. Ross called to me, "Hey, Mom. We're out of mushrooms. Could you go and get us some more?"

"No. Sorry, I'm busy. I've done all I'm going to on the shish-ka-bob."

I heard the door close as someone went out. Then I heard someone else say, "We should have told him to bring more pepper. We're almost out." The door opened and closed again. Music and laughter floated up and I could hear Ross singing. The phone rang; another knock on the door; another greeting.

The party was for a new group of foreign students who had arrived on campus. They were expecting 50 new students from various countries plus all the members of the International Club, and had planned to be outside on the patio. But the weather had turned cold and rainy, so the party had to be moved indoors.

That night, the entire downstairs was jammed—yet, the party seemed not to get off the ground. The Japanese students had to be coaxed to come into the house and were very shy and polite, bowing ceremoniously when introduced to Bill and me. The food was hardly touched, and each nationality seemed to cling together. It was much too quiet, so Bill and I went upstairs to watch television.

A little later, I heard the sound of a guitar and remembered that Scott had left one under the stairs. One of the students from Central America picked it up and started strumming a song which was popular in his country. Soon, someone started singing. Then there was clapping of hands in time with the music. It got louder and louder—so noisy that Bill and I decided to go out and visit friends. When we went downstairs, we saw that they had moved furniture aside and were dancing. The reticent Japanese students smiled and nodded their heads in time with the music.

As Bill and I left, I caught a glimpse of Ross through the crowd, smiling and happily fulfilling his role as host and diplomat.

∾

In April, 1987, Ross walked into the kitchen one Saturday with a bright smile. "Guess what, Mom? My scholarship came through."

"Really? Wonderful. What scholarship?"

"You remember. I told you I had applied for a couple of scholarships to travel to Mexico and Honduras."

"It was such a long time ago, I had forgotten about it. So you got it, did you?"

"One of them is definite, and I'll hear about the other next week, maybe."

"Which one did you get?"

"The one for Honduras the middle of July. But I still want to go with the group to Mexico as soon as school is out. I believe I'll get that one, too."

"What would it cost in case you don't get the scholarship?"

"Not too much—airfare, mainly. They're getting a special discount on that—leaving from New Orleans. They're going to live in a monastery or a nursing home for old people. You have to work to earn your room and board."

"Maybe I can help with the airfare if the scholarship falls through."

"Could you? I'd really like to go. If you can give me any money at all it would help even if I get the scholarship. I'd like to do some things on weekends and visit some of the neighboring areas."

"How did you qualify for the scholarship?" I asked.

"My studies and grades in foreign relations, plus I've got A's in Spanish."

"Can you speak it?"

"No. That's one of the reasons I want to go."

When Bill came in, Ross relayed his news to him.

He said, "I'm proud of you, Ross. That's nice. But I sure do hate to hear that you're planning to go to Honduras. It's pretty unsettled down there. There are lots of problems. You never know when somebody is going to start shooting. You might want to re-think that plan."

"Don't throw cold water on his plans," I said. "He knows about the political climate down there. I trust him. If he wants to go down there and get caught in a cross-fire, let him."

"Thanks, Mom. Thanks a lot. You're not very encouraging, either."

"Is what I think or what your dad might say going to make any difference to you?"

"No, I want to go."

"That's my point. If you've made up your mind, then go for it. Have a good time."

The language classes and the experiences of living among the natives in Mexico helped Ross to attain a passable Spanish speaking ability. He learned to bargain with the street vendors, play games with the children, and communicate with very elderly people in a nursing home. He followed the dietary rules and felt rather smug because he was the only one of the group who hadn't suffered with the often wretched tourist maladies. However, a few days before leaving Merida, he put an ice cube in a drink and within a short time, was hit with stomach cramps.

Bill and I met him at the New Orleans Airport. When the students arrived, Ross was the only one suffering. There was a lot of teasing directed toward him, so I knew he was receiving in return what he had said to them earlier when they were suffering.

He had bought a string hammock for himself, a couple of Mexican shirts for Bill, and pretty embroidered dresses and a necklace for me. The colorful necklace was made of beans. He had bought it from a child.

A week later, he joined the group going to Honduras for six weeks. His stomach problems were still plaguing him when he left but nothing would deter him from making this trip. He was on a roll; he was living his dream.

He stayed with one of the host families and began to feel comfortable with the language. On weekends, the students were free to explore the town and countryside.

When he returned home, we sat at the kitchen table, listening as he related some of the experiences of both trips.

Bill asked him, "What was your overall impression?"

"Poverty. Unbelievable in the twentieth century. I went with this guy and his girlfriend to visit some relatives up in the mountains. It was misty rain that day, which isn't too unusual up in the hills. We hiked up a dirt road for miles, passing shacks with people, chickens, and pigs all living together. The whole family lived in one room."

"Sounds like pictures in *National Geographic.*"

"The children slept on straw mats on the ground but the parents sometimes had a hammock they strung out at night and took down in the morning."

"What sort of food did they eat?"

"I had dinner with the family I visited—beans and bread— their standard meal, three times a day. Sometimes they have eggs. They had this stove they had built on the outside—a piece of sheet metal over an open fire. They fried the beans and bread on it."

"What about the children?" I asked.

"They looked pretty good, considering. They were happy and playing. Their clothes didn't fit, but I noticed a lot of them had American logos on them. Probably came from some charitable organization here."

"Did the parents seem happy?"

"They don't know of any better life. I guess they're happy. The men drink a lot, though. There's not much work for them. They seemed glad I came to visit...happy to share what they had."

Five years had passed since diagnosis in September, 1982. Ross called me from NIH when his tests and examinations were finished. "I'm all clear, Mom."

"Hurray! Wonderful! Five years—Wow!" I said. "What else did you find out? Were you examined? What did they think?"

"They think I'm doing fine. Everything's okay."

"Did they say anything important? What did you talk about with the doctors?"

"The usual."

"No ceremony, no bells ringing? Didn't anybody comment on your five-year anniversary? You must have talked about something important."

"We did—real important. We talked about the economic situation and the needs of the people of Mexico and Honduras," he said. "Really, that's all we talked about."

21

With a little luck and a lot of hard work, it was possible that the fall of 1987 would be the beginning of Ross's senior year at Spring Hill College. He loaded himself up with maximum hours and poured over his work earnestly.

His biggest blow when school began was to learn that Sandra wanted to break up. She had met someone else while he was in Central America. Although he mourned this loss, he threw himself into his studies, and in a few weeks began to date other girls.

James Hutchins and his girl friend, Natalie Kaiser, had proven to be Ross's best friends on campus. James, a sensitive, handsome, and soft-spoken young man with dark, curly hair, had traveled with Ross during the summer and was also studying International Affairs. Another friend, Rebecca Crow—fair-skinned, with long, lustrous red hair—majored in International Marketing. The three of them often studied together.

James, Rebecca, and Ross talked and dreamed for months about an extensive backpacking trip, possibly through Africa, Europe and the Far East. Upon graduation, they planned to find jobs, save every penny, and leave just as soon as they had accumulated enough money to get started. They thought they could finance their trip by working their way through all the countries they wanted to visit. Excitedly, the three of them met, planned, wrote letters, and researched their projected destinations while continuing their studies and final research papers.

Writing term papers had never been as easy for Ross as it had for Mary and Scott, both of whom seemed to enjoy the research, preparation, and creativity required to produce a good paper. Scott's high school papers were still packed away in my collection of memorabilia, along with some of Mary's journalistic endeavors, and her poems.

Ross labored over his term papers to make good grades. One night, after he had finally become satisfied with a paper I had put on the computer disk for him, he announced that he needed a purple tie to wear to class the next day for the oral presentation of his work. I was familiar with his paper on the cultural revolution and new leadership in China, but had no idea why he needed a purple tie.

"I don't think your dad has a purple tie," I said, thinking of Bill's ultra-conservative wardrobe. I stretched my arms and shoulders, yawning as I looked at my watch.

"Please, Mom, help me think where I can find one. Don't you know anybody who might have one I can borrow?"

"I'm not looking for a purple tie at this hour, Ross. I'm tired and need to go home."

"It's important that I have a purple tie for class in the morning, Mom. Can't you please help me?" he whined and pleaded.

"Come on," I said, with exasperation. "Let's get to one of the discount stores before they close."

We rushed into the store and went to the men's clothing section. Quickly, he found a silk tie to his liking but a little loud for my tastes. Just wait until Bill sees this, I thought as Ross drove me home.

The next evening, he told me that he wore his gray pinstriped suit and the purple tie while presenting the paper. He delivered the speech as if he were the new leader of China.

"Why did you have to wear a purple tie?" I asked.

"Because *The Wall Street Journal* reported that the Chairman wore a western pinstriped suit and a bright purple tie when delivering his address to the nation."

He made 100 points on his paper and received 10 extra points for the presentation. He also had a lot of fun.

At the beginning of the winter quarter in January, 1988, Rebecca and Ross founded and became co-editors of the *Spring Hill College Journal of Global Affairs*. Since Ross had worked so hard on his China paper, I think he didn't want it to be forgotten. They collected student writings and, with advice and approval of the faculty, published it. James had contributed an article, and he and Ross worked for hours with the computer specialist on campus, creating a handsome student volume which was later accepted in Spring Hill College's library.

The final rush of finishing papers and taking exams mixed with excitement as graduation neared. Ross didn't want to miss anything connected with graduation, so the seniors' and parents' parties, receptions, and activities kept us busy.

On Saturday, Bill drove to Troy, Alabama, to bring his mother and sister down for the big occasion.

While he was gone, I attended the Baccalaureate on Saturday afternoon in the blazing sun between the historic buildings. Ross filed in with the chorale and I could see sweat rolling down his face as he passed by.

Mary had come home, and that night she joined us at the senior prom at a hotel. Since the graduating class was small compared to most colleges, there were more relatives at the prom than seniors and their dates.

Graduation day was Mother's Day in May, 1988. A clear, cool spring morning greeted us as we gathered on the Avenue of the Oaks for the ceremony. Ross's Grandmother Phelps, aunts, and cousins joined our family under the canopy of oaks, surrounded by dogwood trees and azalea bushes.

Awards were announced and Ross received one for his work on the journal. Then the procession of seniors marched forward to receive their diplomas from the president of the college and the archbishop of the diocese. Ross beamed as he walked toward the podium and gave us a "thumbs up" sign.

When he came back down the aisle carrying his diploma, the sunlight filtered down on him like a blessing. It was a splendid Mother's Day gift.

The rest of Ross's day was spent in saying good-bye to some of his friends. After lunch, Bill left to take his mother and sister back to Troy, while Jean's sons and Mary made several trips to Ross's dorm to move all of his things home. Ross gave instructions that nothing could be touched once it was placed in the house. He wanted to keep all his books and papers. He agreed for Russell and Tosh to take his chairs and carpet for their tree house.

Traditionally, on the night after graduation day, seniors and their friends had returned to the Avenue of the Oaks for their final fling. However, in years past, the party had gotten out of hand with music too loud and too late, noisy singing of rowdy songs, too many party-crashers, and too much beer-drinking, which prompted neighbors to call the police for most of the night. The college president announced, and strongly publicized the fact, that there would be no such party this year. However, through the underground, secret grapevine, word was spread that the party was on. At the appointed time, hundreds of students returned to the Avenue of the Oaks, and the party took place as usual. Reactions, and overreactions, resulted in several students being arrested and spending all or part of the night in jail. Ross was lucky. When I checked the next morning, I found him in bed.

∾

After a few days of rest, Ross concentrated on the big trip that he, James, and Rebecca were going to make. The first step, he decided, was to get in shape physically.

He started jogging every day, often coming into the house soaking wet with sweat, and about to collapse. Whenever I suggested that he take it easy, he reminded me that he had to be very strong physically to do the hiking they had planned.

Within about a week, he came to me one evening and asked, "Mom, what's this bump just below my knee?"

"I don't know what it's called, Ross. Everybody has one." I pointed out the bump under his other knee and on my legs as well.

"Why do you suppose it hurts?" he asked.

I couldn't see swelling anywhere and his legs looked perfectly normal. "What do you expect? You haven't run in years. I'm surprised you're not hurting all over."

Later in the week, he mentioned it again. Again, I didn't pay much attention. I didn't say anything to Bill about it. We were living separate, yet cooperative lives, meeting only when we returned home from work, conversing only about something insignificant and non-controversial.

About two weeks after graduation, Ross, Bill, and I went out to dinner on Friday night. We went by car but decided to stop close by at our friendly neighborhood restaurant where we knew most all the staff and many of their customers.

After Ross strolled around to other tables chatting with friends, he returned to our table and announced that he wasn't very hungry and would settle for a bowl of soup. He was quiet throughout our meal but sat patiently while Bill and I ate.

When we finished, Ross said, "Mom, let's walk home. It's a pretty night and it would be good for you."

"I'm tired, Ross. And I don't have on walking shoes. I don't want to walk home."

"Four blocks? Come on, I think you can handle that."

We left Bill sitting at the table talking to a friend while waiting for the check. We walked along busy Old Shell Road for about two blocks, then turned on Dilston, the short, narrow street which led to ours. There were no cars, so we strolled down the middle of the tree-lined street. A jogger sprinted past and we greeted others who were outside walking in the crystal clear, late spring evening. Ross paused to pat the head of a friendly dog.

As I looked up through the overhanging limbs of the oak trees, I saw stars in a dark blue-gray sky. I reflected on the splendid conclusion of this chapter of Ross's life.

Strolling slowly along, Ross put his arm around my shoulder and said, "Mom, I hate to tell you, but I've got some bad news."

Expecting some tale of woe about a college friend or a bad dent in the car, or perhaps some unexpected expense he hadn't told me about, I asked, "What's up? Let's have it."

"I went to see Dr. Daugherty."

"What for?" I asked, whirling around to face him.

"I've got a tumor in my leg."

I stopped walking. "You've what? What did you say?"

"I've got a tumor in my leg. That's why it's been hurting."

Silently, we stared at each other.

"The hell you have! What do you mean? What are you talking about?"

He laughed at my outburst. "Calm down, Mom. Just calm down...."

I took several deep breaths and said, "That...makes...me...so...damn...mad! I don't believe it. Whoever heard of such a thing!"

"Don't talk so loud, Mom. Just calm down." He tilted his head backward and laughed again.

I turned to face him. "Ross, don't do me this way. Tell me everything. How do you know? Are you sure? Did you see the X-ray? When did you see Dr. Daugherty?"

"I saw him yesterday and I saw the X-ray. It looks sort of like it did before. But I don't think it's as big or broken out of the bone. He told me to go to the Infirmary tomorrow for a CT scan."

"I don't believe this. You've had bone scans. How long has it been since you had a bone scan? When were you at NIH last?"

"I don't know—last year—I can't remember when."

"It cannot be, Ross. What did the doctor say?"

"He didn't say much. He thinks it's osteo. That's why I have to get a CT."

"It *cannot* be osteo! It's been six years. It's got to be something else. Have you talked to anybody at NIH?"

"No, no...not yet. There's no point until after the scan."

We walked a few slow steps past a neighbor who sat on his front porch. "Lovely evening, isn't it?" he called to us.

"Yes...yes, it is." I lowered my voice and said to Ross, "I want to talk to Dr. Daugherty."

"No, you can't. Not yet, Mom. Let me handle it. You can talk to him later if you want to. You can't talk to anybody until after the CT scan. Promise?"

I couldn't promise.

He continued to chuckle and slowly shake his head, recalling my reaction. He seemed relieved that I didn't burst into tears.

Suddenly, the evening felt dark and cold. I held Ross's arm for support as we continued sauntering toward our house. He turned his head toward me slightly and looked at me out of the corner of his eye.

"I'll be all right, Ross. Give me a little time. This is hard to take."

"Believe me, I know."

Three noisy adolescents whizzed by on their bikes, full of energy and high spirits to be out in the street after dark. In the far distance, I heard the evening train as it blew its whistle at the crossing. Crickets chirped.

"Mom, I've thought a lot about it, and I want you to promise me three things. Okay? You've got to promise."

"What three things?"

"I don't want you to quit your job. I want you to make Dad get involved this time. And I don't want it to split the family apart like it did before."

"Your problems didn't split the family apart. They didn't create any new problems in our family, Ross. They could have brought to the surface some old problems that were already there, but what happened to you didn't cause our problems. As for getting your dad more involved, you'll have to talk to him yourself."

For the next few steps, he said nothing.

"Have you told your dad?"

"No, not yet."

"Well, when are you going to tell him?"

"I don't know...I don't know."

"You've got to tell him, Ross."

"I know...."

Bill drove past us as we continued toward our driveway.

PART THREE

June, 1988—October, 1989

22

June, 1988

In the near darkness of our front yard, Ross paced slowly around, then stopped and leaned his back against a tree. He softly called and greeted the cats.

When I entered the house, I saw Bill sitting in the den watching television. When Ross walked in with Maggie draped across his shoulder, I listened for him to tell his dad about the new problem, but he said nothing. Although it was still early evening, I went upstairs, went to bed, and buried my head under a pillow.

Whenever possible, Ross slept in the mornings as late as he could. This Saturday morning, however, he was up early, showered and dressed before coming downstairs.

"What are you doing up so early?" Bill asked. "Are you going somewhere?"

"Yes."

"Where you off to? Where you going?"

"Out."

"What's the big deal? Can't you say where you're going?"

"The Mobile Infirmary."

"The Infirmary? What for?"

"To get a CT scan," he said, as he walked out the door.

Bill shrugged his shoulders and turned to me. "What was that all about?"

"Dr. Daugherty found a tumor in his leg."

His shoulders slumped as he stood staring at me. "When?"

"Thursday."

"Where?"

"In his right leg, below the knee."

He heaved a sigh, turned and left the room with no comment.

I went out and sat on the patio, coffee cup in hand. A kitten jumped up in my lap and another curled itself around my ankles. Blue jays squawked and tiny little sparrows twittered higher in the trees. I listened for the haunting, gentle call of the mourning dove.

...It could be something other than osteo—something benign. From the moment Ross had decided it was time to visit Dr. Daugherty until he got up the courage to tell me, I hadn't noticed any difference in his mood or behavior. Even when he told me, he expressed no fear or sadness. He matter-of-factly stated the circumstances, taking one step at a time.

He was gone for a long time—at least, it seemed so. Perhaps he had decided not to come home. Maybe he drove past the Infirmary without stopping.

In a couple of hours, I heard his car pull into the driveway. He sauntered onto the patio, and the cats moved to meet him. He picked them up—one on his shoulder with its hind legs hanging down his back, and the other under his arm.

"When will you know?" I asked.

"Not till Monday. I have an appointment with Dr. Daugherty at two-fifteen."

"Did the technicians say anything? Was there a doctor there?"

"No, Mom. I'm not going to discuss it anymore until I see Dr. Daugherty."

"I told your dad."

"What did he say?"

"Nothing."

He walked around the back of the house to find Bill. After a few minutes, he went upstairs to his bedroom and closed the door.

Waiting had begun again. Sunday was a day to get through, to muddle along, hour by hour. Late in the afternoon, Ross and I again sat on the patio.

"You know, Mom, you could really improve the looks of our yard. Why don't you plant lots of flowers out here?"

"We have too much shade and too many tree roots. I've tried it many times. Between those problems and the different dogs we've had, I gave up trying to have something blooming."

"Don't ever give up, Mom. We should have put a fish pond and a fountain out here a long time ago."

"Your dad never wanted a fountain. He has an aversion to cement statuary. He puts it in the same category as plastic pink flamingoes."

"We could make a fountain out of rocks—natural looking—and the water could fall into a fish pond."

"I'm too tired to start big projects. My job takes most of my hours and energy."

"Maybe you give too much of yourself to your job, Mom. Do you really like it that much?"

"It's a unique job and I'm lucky to have it."

"Why don't you do something else sometime—something for yourself, something you would enjoy? Why don't you go back to school and work on your degree? *Stop putting off things you want to do with your life.*"

"I'm too tired for evening classes. Maybe later."

"What are you going to do for vacation this year?"

"I don't know yet. Let's wait and see."

"Remember what you promised, Mom. You're not going to quit your job."

"I didn't promise that. Let's wait and see."

"I'm not a kid anymore. You don't have to give up your job like you did before."

"I'll agree to talk to Mr. Callahan about it, but that's all I promise. So let's drop that subject, okay?"

"Okay, but don't make any big decision without discussing it with me. I'll tell you when I need you. I mean it, Mom! Don't quit your job until you check with me."

"I'd like to go with you to see the doctor tomorrow."

"No, Mom. It's not necessary," he sighed with exasperation. "I told you to let me handle it. Okay?"

Monday afternoon, he phoned me at my office. Dr. Daugherty had told him that indications pointed to osteosarcoma. All the signs were there. He told Ross to go immediately to NIH. The appointment had already been made and he was to leave the next day. When I asked if I could go with him, he said, "No."

When he flew up to Washington for his appointment at NIH, he had to change planes in Nashville. Upon re-boarding, he was pleasantly surprised to see Rebecca Crow already seated on the plane. She was on her way to Washington for some interviews. They managed to plan sightseeing excursions in between their scheduled appointments.

When Ross telephoned me, he said there were a few familiar staff members at the desk in the clinic but all the Clinical Associates were total strangers. He asked his doctor to call me at work.

When the young man called, he said that examination and consultation indicated that it was osteosarcoma. He would have to research Ross's previous records, and he promised to keep me informed. When he called again on Friday, he said that Ross had met with radiologists and surgeons. He was vague and would only say, "Ross has presented a very 'knotty' problem." Further X-rays had been ordered and Ross had to stay through the weekend for the Monday appointment.

Rebecca remained in Washington until Sunday, and the two of them walked miles and talked for hours. Their planned backpack expedition was uppermost in their minds. They had worked on the details of their trip for a year.

During the weekend, I visited the Maysons on their patio and discussed their fountain. Their next-door neighbor also had one and we walked over to look at it. Later in the day, I drove to nurseries and places which sold fountains and statuary. The urgency in getting a fountain and fish pond in place propelled me from place to place. After driving aimlessly around town on often unfamiliar streets, I jerked myself back to the present, and decided to postpone plans for a pond and fountain.

Ross had planned to be at Camp Rap-A-Hope this week and

he called the director from Bethesda to let her know he would be late arriving. He had X-rays on Monday and was told to return home and wait for their call.

Back in Mobile, he joined the counselors and campers at Camp Rap-A-Hope. Word had gotten around about his condition, and staff members were saddened at the news. Ross had been their shining example for the little campers who were struggling through their treatment. He stayed at the camp until it ended on Saturday, but he told me he had spent a lot of time alone in the woods and by the lake.

His case had been presented to the Tumor Board at NIH on Monday night, but no one called with a consensus of opinion.

The next day, I walked into the Congressman's office and closed the door behind me. In this election year, he had strong opposition and the work load in the congressional office had increased correspondingly. However, after we discussed Ross's new development, he assured me that I should plan to do whatever I had to do. I would still have my job.

When Ross's doctor telephoned me at work the following Friday, he gave the collective opinion of all involved: It appeared to be osteosarcoma and a biopsy was scheduled for June 23rd. He found answers to my questions if he could, and called me back. He said that Ross appeared to be a good candidate for a limb-sparing procedure. The surgical specialist from September, 1982, was still around. Dr. Martin Malawer had a private practice in Washington and also worked with NIH. Before Ross was released to return to Mobile, he was told that he might be Dr. Malawer's third patient at NIH for this type surgery.

23

Ross and I flew back to Washington National Airport the following week, and after collecting our luggage, we walked through the rushing crowds past the line of people waiting on the sidewalk for a cab. On the other side of a long row of taxis stood the shelter for the NIH shuttle, and I hoped we hadn't missed its hourly run.

We watched the hurrying people, the traffic, and confusion for a few minutes. When the bus arrived, we settled back for the speedy—sometimes harrowing—ride along the Potomac River toward Maryland.

When we reached the Clinic Center, it seemed as if the past five years hadn't happened. But something was different. The crowds and noise were missing. Only two or three people sat on benches in front of the entrance. I didn't see a taxi, a shuttle bus, an ambulance, or a line of cars waiting to collect or discharge passengers. Inside the lobby, only a few people moved about. We deposited our luggage in the same unlocked cabinet we had used so many times during 1982 and 1983.

As we walked past the transportation desk, I saw the first familiar faces. The same three men were still sitting there. The private travel office had different personnel, but they still sat at their computers and had phones to their ears.

Ross had a chest X-ray and EKG that afternoon. Afterwards, we went to our hotel—the only one we could find in the area with a room available. It lacked warmth and offered little comfort. We tried to have dinner in the coffee shop, but neither of us had an appetite. Ross, locked in his own thoughts, sat silently at the table.

He spent most of the next day in the Physical Therapy Department getting precise measurements of his leg. While the therapists watched and took notes, he squatted, rose to his tip-toes, and walked on ramps and stairs.

That evening, he went to the admissions desk to enter the hospital. Again, he was assigned to Pediatrics, which had been moved to the 13th floor. As we walked through the gallery on our way to the elevator, I paused to look at the art work on the walls—soft pastels in an almost surrealistic style. Classical music played softly on the speakers. The old, cheerless furniture had been replaced with bright sectional modules arranged in conversational areas. The elevators hadn't been improved. The waiting was still interminable.

When we reached the 13th floor, we learned that the admitting office had made an error in sending Ross there. All beds were previously committed, and the overflow had to go to the 12th floor. Taking our luggage, we returned to the elevator.

In his room on the 12th floor, his nurse entered wearing a Public Health Service uniform which looked military and somehow intimidating. Although Ross didn't have a roommate yet, she told me I couldn't stay in the room with him at night. More important things were on her mind. When she tried to draw blood, she found that his veins had not recovered from the chemotherapy five years before.

After she left, Dr. Malawer, the surgeon we had heard about for so many years, came in to see Ross for the first time.

He had a lilting voice with a slight foreign accent. A handsome man with olive skin and dark brown eyes, he smiled as he reached to shake Ross's hand. Although he moved around very fast, he spoke slowly and softly. He explained that he would design the limb-sparing procedure, and he wanted nothing done which might interfere with his overall plan. He didn't go into detail about the operation, but the biopsy, scheduled for 7:30 the next morning, would be done by him personally. After the doctor left us, I gathered my luggage and returned to the hotel.

When I arrived in Ross's room early the next morning, the attendants brought a gurney to his bedside and he crawled over onto it. At the swinging double door on the surgery floor, I kissed him on his forehead. I stood there in the hall for a few minutes, leaning against the wall. People in white coats passed hurriedly through the swinging door. I looked through the glass panel, and far along the hall, I could see Ross and his attendant. When they moved out of sight around a corner, I returned to the elevator and went to the first floor.

Outside the cafeteria, mobs of workers were arriving just as I remembered from years before. Several different languages punctuated the air. Something had damaged the grass, and new footpaths criss-crossed the lawn. Pieces of paper and debris blew around. I wondered what had happened to the vegetable garden which the staff had carefully tended in one of the flower beds in 1983.

As I sat on a bench under the trees, I saw one of Ross's favorite nurses from 1982 and 1983. I rose to speak to her, but she only glanced at me—not remembering. I returned to the bench and continued to search the faces as they passed.

When I returned to the waiting room, I learned that the biopsy was finished and Ross would soon be in his room. His nurse said he could have pain medication, but he had to request it. It couldn't be given automatically. He asked for it.

In the evening when Ross was fully awake, Dr. Malawer came in to discuss the proposed surgical procedure. He drew a rough sketch showing that they would remove his knee and one and a half inches of the femur, plus seven inches of the tibia—six inches both ways from the tumor. An implant—an internal prosthesis—would be placed in his leg. The prosthesis, to be especially designed and manufactured for Ross, would take several weeks.

Dr. Malawer leaned back in his chair and said, "Ross, I've had plans for many months to be out of the country in August. I don't want to operate on you and then leave town. I would like to postpone your surgery until I return in September. I cannot delay this trip—I'm sorry."

"That's a long time," Ross said. "How many weeks are you talking about?"

"About twelve," he said.

Twelve weeks of waiting and wondering what changes were going on in the tumor. We both knew the only other alternative. Although Ross and I hadn't discussed it, I would encourage him to refuse amputation and take his chances on chemotherapy alone if nothing could be done surgically. But it would have to be his decision.

"Do you need to think about it?" Dr. Malawer asked.

"No," Ross said. "I'll wait."

"Okay. I'm very particular about casts. In a few days, I want you to go to Children's Hospital to have one put on. My associates there know exactly what I want and how I want it done. I don't want anyone else putting a cast on your leg. You will also need angiograms which I want done at Children's."

We didn't question this, but 12 weeks later, I would be vividly reminded of his statement about the cast.

He called for a brace and ordered Ross to keep it on at all times. While waiting for the cast, he had to be extremely careful because the worst thing that could happen would be to break the weakened bone in his leg. In that event, the planned surgery couldn't take place.

Instead of waiting 12 weeks doing nothing, the oncologists and surgeons agreed that chemotherapy should begin as soon as he recuperated from the biopsy.

The next day, Ross went by wheelchair to the Physical Therapy Department, where a special crutch was assembled for his left arm. It had an elbow rest with a device to be placed in the hook of his prosthesis. There were straps to go around the prosthesis, which fastened to the crutch with Velcro tape. In spite of the weakness of the upper left arm, it worked.

When Ross was discharged from the hospital, we checked into the Marriott Hotel. I was thankful I had my own funds and credit card. Bill must have been thankful for that fact, too. The Marriott gave a big discount on the rooms to NIH patients, and Ross received a stipend for being a part of a study, but even so, it wouldn't take long to run up a big hotel bill.

The Marriott gave us our usual spacious handicapped room on the first floor which had recently been completely redecorated in soft greens, ivory, and pale yellow. I opened the drapes and the sliding glass door, and pulled a lounge chair onto our little terrace overlooking the pool. Ross sat with his leg elevated, listening to music on his small tape player.

In the evening, we had dinner in the Bello Mondo and found it as pleasant as we had remembered. Ross chose his favorite—fettuccine Alfredo—but he didn't finish it. He didn't seem to be in any hurry to leave the restaurant. Yet he remained silent, picking at his dessert—not looking at me. We listened to the Italian music and tried to guess the names of familiar operatic compositions.

"I think I'll go on to the room," he said.

"Want me to go with you? I'm finished."

"No, take your time. Drink your coffee. Enjoy the music."

"You okay?" I asked.

"I'm okay."

He stood and fastened the crutch to his prosthesis. I watched as he maneuvered the two steps down from our seating area, recalling that crutches on carpet could be treacherous.

I lingered until the waiter showed impatience. Then I wandered into the lobby and gift shop, killing time.

When I returned to the room, the drapes were closed and Ross had his face buried in a pillow. Tissues were scattered on the floor. He cleared his throat and swallowed hard. "Could you find some place to go, Mom? Just for a little while?"

"Sure...I'll see you later."

I walked outside the hotel, through the parking lots, then sat at a table near the pool. Joggers returned from their workouts, cooling down and mopping their heads with towels. Moms and dads and children on vacation released pent-up energy in the water.

About an hour later, I re-entered the room and found Ross sitting in bed, propped up on a pillow. His shirt and prosthesis lay beside him, the crutches on the floor. He stared at the television.

"I'm sorry, Ross, but I need to go to bed. I'm very tired."

"Don't worry about it. Could you turn the volume up? The remote doesn't work for volume—just On, Off and Channels."

"Okay. Anything else?"

"Could you get me a Pepsi from the machine? And if the gift shop is still open, I'd like to have a *TV Guide*."

After I poured his drink over ice cubes, I began to straighten the room. "Do you want me to help you hop to the bathroom before I go to bed?"

"No, I'll manage."

"Not in the dark, you can't. Wake me before you try it."

"No, I won't. I told you I can manage."

"Need anything else?"

"You can put a couple of pillows under my leg, and my pills and a glass of water where I can reach them. Is the TV going to bother you?"

"Maybe...for at least two minutes."

As I walked into the bathroom, I cleared a path, moving shoes, bags, and other items from the floor. After I brushed my teeth and washed my face, I moved the bath mat out of the way and placed a towel and cloth on the counter with Ross's toiletries beside them. Finally, I crawled onto the far side of my bed, faced the wall, and put a pillow over my head.

"Can you do without the light?" I mumbled.

"In a few minutes."

"Aren't you sleepy yet?"

"No, try to go to sleep."

"Goodnight. I love you, Ross."

"Goodnight. Love you, too. And Mom...?"

"Hmm?"

"I'm sorry you have to go through this again."

The trip to Children's Hospital for the angiogram on Monday took the whole day. Through a mixup in communication with NIH, they admitted Ross. When everything finally got straightened out, he spent the entire day on a gurney in the hall of the laboratory section. We returned to the hotel at 8:00 p.m.

He hardly slept that night. I could hear him in the dark as he cleared his throat and blew his nose. I heard the clicks of the prosthesis as he adjusted it to fit the crutch before going into the bathroom.

That same night, the Tumor Board at NIH again reviewed his case, although they didn't have the final pathology report. Again, their preliminary conclusion: osteosarcoma.

The next day, he had an appointment with a member of the NIH staff we hadn't met before. Jacques Bolle, a psychiatric nurse, worked with patients throughout the hospital, and he told Ross he had arranged an appointment for him with a private counselor in Chevy Chase.

While Ross met with Jacques, I wanted to talk with the doctors. Dr. Philip Pizzo still held the title of Chief Oncologist, Pediatric Branch. Dr. Marc Horowitz had recently come to NIH from St. Jude's in Tennessee and served as Outpatient Clinical Director of Pediatrics.

I had already questioned several associates and learned of disagreements among them as to what Ross's new development meant. One group believed the problem was a metastasis of the original tumor. The other side said it could not be.

Often, they said, "It's not unheard of." I heard the expression so many times that I concluded that they had agreed among themselves that, when worse came to worst with my questions, they could always say, "It's not unheard of."

I cornered one of the young doctors in the hall. "Where can I find information on previous cases like this?" I asked.

With a soft, southern drawl, he said, "I'm not positive, but I seem to recall hearing of a similar case when I was in medical school." He also pointed out something I had already learned: It occasionally happens that two different types of cancer are discovered at the same time.

From 1982, I remembered a case on the 10th surgery floor. A beauty contest winner, a 20-year-old girl with an operatic voice, had been sent to NIH following a radical mastectomy. After the surgery on her breast, they found bone cancer in her shoulder.

I saw Dr. Poplack in the cafeteria. A quiet and unassuming man, I remembered his soft voice from years ago as he spoke to us when the group of doctors made rounds in the evening. I had heard that he believed Ross's problem was a metastasis, and, when I asked him, he said, "It has to be. There can be no other explanation."

"But what if it's not? What does this mean?" I asked.

With a perplexed look on his face, he said, "Do you realize what a Pandora's box would be opened if it's not a metastasis? Would we be admitting there is something in Ross's system and bones that produces sarcomas?"

While Dr. Horowitz tried to be non-committal, I had the feeling that he thought differently. I spied him through the crowd in the downstairs lobby and worked my way over to him to ask for a moment of his time.

"Let's talk now," he said, as he took my arm and ushered me to a private spot in the gallery. We stood behind a column and he leaned his tall frame against it. His tie was loosened, and his unruly dark hair had fallen across his forehead.

"What can you tell me about Ross's new problem? What happened? What does this mean?"

"I can't tell you much more than you've already been told. Ross has presented a challenge. We honestly don't know—we're just not that smart," he said, as he rubbed his forehead with his fingertips and ran his hand through his hair.

"Dr. Poplack thinks it's a metastasis from the original site in his wrist," I said.

"He may be right, but I can't quite buy that."

"Why didn't it show up before? Why, after six years, does it suddenly appear?"

He looked away toward a distant door and said, "Actually, it didn't 'suddenly appear.' It showed up on some of his old X-rays."

"What? What do you mean? Why wasn't it addressed when it was discovered?" I asked, my mind reeling.

He quickly leaned toward me, his hand on my shoulder. "Wait a minute, now. There's never a one-hundred-percent totally clear, unblemished picture. Many things can cause a shadow on the film. No one suspected a tumor in his leg and the shadow was thought to be insignificant. If we had to check out every tiny mark on every X-ray, there would be no end to it."

"Someone has been negligent," I said.

He shook his head from side to side. "No one has been negligent. The X-rays and CTs of his chest have been watched carefully. That's where we expect to find a metastasis and it's also part of the reason I don't think this is one. Even if it could be proven that it was there as long as two years ago, too much time would have passed for me to believe it was a spread of the original tumor. Remember, if osteo spreads, you can bet it will happen during the first two years."

I had heard this statement many times before. "I remember from the protocol sheet that one of the drugs could cause second malignancies. Could that be it?"

"We don't think so. The second malignancies referred to are most often associated with leukemia. But, Mrs. Phelps, what choice was there at the time? We did what we thought best."

"What kind of treatment do you plan? Can he take any of the drugs he had before?"

"Some of them—no. He's had his limit. Others—possibly. But on the outside chance that this is a metastasis, why would we want to? If the drugs weren't effective in eradicating the cells the first time, why try again? We'll try different drugs."

"Are there any new ones?"

"Yes, the protocol for relapse of osteosarcoma calls for two drugs, Ifosfamide and VP 16. That's what we plan for Ross."

"I thought you said you didn't believe it was a relapse."

"Mrs. Phelps," he said wearily. "What difference does it make whether it is or not? The point is, the problem is here and must be addressed. It really doesn't help to debate why or where it came from. We have no other treatment protocol. This is all there is."

He remained silent as I shielded my eyes with my hand and stared at the floor. This is all there is...this is all there is. "Thanks for your honesty. I'll probably be looking for you again with more questions."

"Anytime. I'm here whenever you need me," he said. He squeezed my shoulder before he dashed for the elevator, his head and shoulders several inches ahead of the rest of his body.

24

As I wandered around the reception area, I glanced up at the big black clock on the wall, its hour hand on 4:00 p.m. Ross's appointment at 4:30 with the counselor was in Chevy Chase—seven miles away. I considered telephoning his office to postpone the appointment, but remembered Ross's emphatic instructions that I was not to intrude in any way. I slowly paced the hall, silently repeating the fact that the growth, or whatever it was, in Ross's leg could be benign. Some people receive that blessed report. Maybe it's something harmless—something that will go away. Maybe he can still go backpacking.

Near the elevator, I looked left and right through the moving crowd searching for any familiar faces, but there were none. When I spotted Ross struggling the block-long hike from the elevator to the front entrance, I caught up with him.

"I've called a taxi," I said to him.

"Why? There's no need for a taxi. Let's ride the metro," he said, as he slowed to catch his breath.

"No, Ross. It would be too risky. Remember what Malawer said about the danger of breaking your leg? The brace isn't that strong."

"There's no danger in riding the metro. I'm not going in a taxi." Although his eyes were bright, he was pale. Perspiration oozed around the edges of the hair on his forehead.

"I'm not afraid of the metro. The escalator is the problem. We're not taking any chances. We'll take a taxi."

The clock on the wall revealed that I had won the argument by default. We didn't have time to ride the shuttle to the metro and make his appointment. He reluctantly got into the cab. Our driver only pretended to understand English, smiling and nodding at everything we said. Ross tried to talk with him. When he figured out that the driver had recently arrived from Africa, he whispered to me to be patient. Ross pointed out where to turn or which lane to get in. The driver said, *"Yas, yas."*

After a few backups and turnarounds, Ross spotted the building and, even though we were on the wrong side of the street, he told the driver to stop. We got out of the cab, and I looked across six lanes packed with speeding vehicles. We approached the curb and waited with other pedestrians for the "walk" lights.

With his unbending right knee and weak left shoulder, Ross gripped the crutches and sailed into the street as he called, "Come on, Mom! Let's go!"

I chased close behind, and watched as he eyed the pavement, swinging his right leg and hopping on his left foot. When we reached the island halfway across the intersection, the light changed again. He caught his breath and balanced for a moment, the right crutch under his arm. He opened and closed his right hand, stretching his fingers and wiping sweat on his pants leg. I handed him a tissue to dry his brow.

Traffic sped past on both sides, whipping dust and debris around us as we stood on the narrow neutral ground. When the light changed again, I stepped ahead of him, silently daring anyone to move until he got across. I pretended to ignore the impatient stares and beeping horns. Ross's silent message reached me: "Don't make a scene, Mom, don't make a scene."

When we found the building, we rode the elevator to the second floor. While Ross met with the counselor, I walked along the hall to a Mexican restaurant. Sitting at a table on the balcony terrace, I ordered a cup of coffee. It was too early for dinner guests and there were only two other customers, reading newspapers and drinking beer.

Except for muffled traffic noises, it was quiet on the terrace—a welcome respite from a hectic day. I leaned back in my chair and listened to a melancholy arrangement of *Sorrento* drifting from the sound system. I'd been fairly successful all day in keeping at bay the unutterable feelings surrounding the first diagnosis almost six years ago. But now, in this moment of relative stillness, I began to sense a weakening. Quickly, I got up, put on my dark glasses, and strolled along the wall of the terrace, studying the exotic plants.

When Ross finished his session, he hobbled out to the terrace and reminded me he had not had time for lunch. While still standing, he stopped a waiter and ordered a burrito and a Mexican beer. Then he placed his crutches on a chair and hopped around to sit beside me so he could watch the passers-by.

When he finished eating, he said, "Let's ride the metro back."

"No, Ross," I sighed. "Let's don't go through that again."

"Look down at the street, Mom. You couldn't get a cab for hours. It's after five o'clock. I'm not going to wait around for a taxi."

From where I sat, I could see Wisconsin Avenue and one of the side streets which led into it. Traffic had come to a standstill. "All right," I mumbled.

We had entered the building by an elevator, and I rose to move in that direction. Ross headed for a short escalator directly in front of us. Restaurant patrons and a few office workers were moving up and down.

At street level, the escalator emptied onto a concrete-paved promenade leading to the metro. After watching and plotting for a few minutes, Ross got on. Right before he reached the end, he started to fall and dropped his right crutch. The left crutch, still fastened to the prosthesis, went down with him as he fell backward on the landing. His braced right leg pointed up in the air; his left arm, prosthesis, and crutch were askew.

An elderly man stepped forward, helped him to get up, and said, "I'm sorry I wasn't closer. I could have caught you before you hit the ground."

"It's all right," Ross said. "I'm okay."

"You sure? Can I help you with anything?"

Ross shook his head. He glanced at the 5:00 crowd of commuters hurrying by, craning their necks, staring at the confusion. He clenched his teeth, swore softly, and looked at me with fury in his eyes.

"Did you hurt your leg?" I asked, reaching toward him.

He jerked back. "No! Leave me alone, will you?"

"Let me help you get the crutch fastened," I said.

"Will you please leave me alone and get out of my way!" He tugged at the entangled Velcro tape.

I turned away and nodded a thanks to the gentleman who had tried to help. I saw compassion in his eyes as he turned and left.

Looking back at Ross, I said, "That does it—I don't care if we stay here all night. I'm getting a taxi and I don't want to hear another word about it."

"Go ahead and try. See if you can get one. You'll see."

I stalked off to the nearest corner, leaving him standing there fuming. I craned my neck, stood on my tiptoes, waved my hand, and yelled, "Taxi!" As I walked toward the next corner, I stopped to tap on windshields. The drivers wouldn't even look at me. Half-way around the block, I began to admit defeat. I plodded on until I spied Ross where he waited, crutches and prosthesis in place. I cautiously approached him.

"You're right. I give up. Let's look for the elevator for the train. There has to be one around here somewhere."

"The escalator is right over there, Mom. I'm not looking for the elevator. I'm riding the damn escalator!"

"All right, hard head. Go ahead. Break your leg...Or maybe your neck. Be a jerk!"

"Just don't forget, Mom. It's my leg and my neck."

Tight-lipped, silent, we approached the escalator. The steps went so deep into the cavernous darkness that we couldn't see the end of it. People dodged around each other, loaded down with briefcases and shopping bags, as they rushed to get on.

Ross stood and watched for a few minutes, then approached the moving stairs. "Stand behind me, Mom. If I start to fall, just hold me until I get my balance."

"Sure, Ross, sure. You bet. Fall backward, please."

Cautiously, he placed his right crutch on the first step. The moving stair step quickly folded and he realized that he couldn't hop on with one foot. He let go of the crutch and it bounced and clanged on down the escalator with us still standing at the top.

I closed my eyes.

"You've got to do something, Mom. Don't just stand there shaking your head!"

"Grab something and hold on," I called, as I quickly stepped on and started down. "And stay right there! Don't you move."

"Just where do you think I could go, Mom? How do you think I could move?" he called after me.

I worked my way down around the other riders and, at the bottom of the escalator, I saw a bewildered-looking man holding the crutch, his eyes scanning the crowd. I rushed up to him.

"Sir...Sir...That's mine," I said. "I mean, it's my son's. He's up there." I pointed to the top of the stairs.

"Hope he's not hurt, lady. These things can be dangerous flying through the air, you know."

"No, he's not hurt. He's okay—and thanks," I said. I took the crutch and joined the up-moving line. I kept my eyes on my feet and by the time I reached the top, I was resigned.

"What now?" I asked, when I found Ross.

"I've got it figured out. I can do it. Just listen and I'll tell you what to do."

I didn't argue.

"Listen carefully. Pay attention to what I tell you. I'll unfasten the Velcro, take the left crutch off, and hand it to you. Then, just before I hop on, I'll hand you the right one. You hold both of them while I grab the hand rail. When I hop on, you jump on right behind me with the crutches."

"Then? What happens next? What do we do when we get to the bottom?"

"When I get on, you hop on real quick. Get right behind me and stay until I get my balance. Then you hurry and get in front of me. Go on down a few steps so that when I reach the bottom, you can be waiting, holding the crutches when I hop off."

"What happens if I'm not ready for you to jump off? What if I can't get down fast enough and have the crutches in place?"

"You can if you do what I say. Can't you at least try?"

"I don't want to think about it. Let's get it over with."

We waited for a lull in the horde of people who rushed to get on. Nearby traffic roared, people bumped into each other.

Ross loosened the straps and handed me the left crutch. Seconds passed as he stared intently for the right instant to make his move. Suddenly, he tossed the right crutch to me, grabbed the hand rail, and hopped on with his left foot, swaying, then balancing. "Jump on, Mom! Hurry! You've got to catch me if I fall!"

Sure, I thought, as I struggled with briefcase, purse, and two unwieldy crutches. "Stop looking back at me!" I yelled. "Hold on!" I lurched onto the top step, wobbled, and almost fell.

"Get ready," Ross called over his shoulder. "Hurry! You've got to move ahead of me."

Awkwardly, I stepped down around him. A bottleneck of passengers blocked me.

"Excuse me," I called. "I've got to get through. Let me pass, please...Sorry, I've got to pass...." I tried to smile at those who looked with suspicion at the curious spectacle.

The escalators created a roaring wind tunnel; the speeding trains at the lower level thundered to their stops.

At the bottom of the escalator, I tossed my purse and briefcase on the floor and got the crutches in position. When I looked up, I saw Ross riding down, smiling and nonchalantly chatting with another passenger as if he did this daily.

Still smiling, he confidently hopped off, grabbed me by the shoulder to steady himself, and took his left crutch. With my arm around his waist, he calmly refastened the straps to the prosthesis then took the right crutch.

"Nothing to it," he said. "Let's get our tickets."

Without a word to each other, we repeated the performance on the escalator down to the train level. Even on the train, we didn't speak.

When we arrived at the Medical Center station and started walking toward the exit, I stopped and turned to him. "If you say one word about riding the escalator, I'll walk off and leave you. Do you understand?"

"Okay, okay, we'll take the elevator," he laughed. "I just wanted to prove I could do it."

∾

The next day, he had to return to Children's Hospital to have a heavy cast put on his leg from hip to ankle. After he practiced on the crutches with the added weight of the cast, we rushed back to our hotel to gather our luggage and catch the shuttle to National Airport for our return trip to Mobile.

I stared out the window of the shuttle as it passed through the Virginia countryside along the Potomac River. A feeling of guilt arose when I remembered that I still hadn't complimented Ross or said, "Congratulations! You rode the escalator!" or something. I couldn't recall anyone saying anything encouraging to him since we'd arrived in Bethesda. He deserved better—a pat on the back, applause, even a trophy. Anything would have been better than my impatience and anger.

But the moment passed and I didn't bring up the subject again. Time—there was never enough time to linger over any one incident because another appeared, and then another, an even greater contest.

When the shuttle arrived at the airport, after I unloaded luggage and got the crutches in place, Ross went through the gymnastics of getting out of the van. He stepped out into dry, hot wind which whipped through a porte cochere where cars, taxis, and vans waited their turn. A policeman twirled around, hands raised, blowing his whistle and shouting at drivers and pedestrians. Sirens, car engines, beeping horns, yells from drivers and skycaps muffled the roar of nearby metro trains.

Ross held our place in line while I pushed our luggage toward the ticket counter. At last, we received our tickets and wove our way through the crowd toward the security gate.

Old memories flooded over me again when Ross approached the checkpoint—all those times when he was embarrassed because of having to unbutton his shirt in front of strangers so the guards could make a closer inspection of the straps, cables, and buckles holding his prosthesis in place.

Before he even began to walk through the security gate, two uniformed men rose with their two-way radios and moved toward him. They stepped outside the barrier, scanned him, hand-frisked him, and asked questions about his prosthesis and crutches. They looked under his shirt and scanned the cast on his leg. He turned his head away when people stared and looked back at him with curiosity or suspicion or both.

A big, burly, black man in a black uniform, carrying a black billy club stepped forward in an authoritative manner. What now? I wondered.

With a surprisingly soft voice, the man asked, "Are you a patient at the National Cancer Institute?"

"Yes, I am," Ross said softly, as he stared at the floor.

The man stepped back, bowed low, and with a flourish of his arms said, "Then walk right through, brother. God be with you! Go for it, man, go for it!"

As we walked toward the departure gate, we looked back at him through the crowd, and though my vision had clouded, I saw that he was still watching us.

He raised both arms high above his head and formed the victory sign with his fingers. He called in a loud voice, "Good luck, my man, good luck!"

25

July, 1988

Once he finally got on the plane, Ross's stiff leg made it impossible for him to sit in his assigned seat. They gave him a seat in the first-class section, placing the crutches in the closet. When I took my seat, an attendant asked me to move to the front to be with him.

As soon as I sat down and fastened my seat belt, he said, "I need you to help me think of something I can do. I don't want to be just a patient. I've got to do something else. Try to think of something."

"Are you thinking of work, or maybe going to school?"

"I don't know what I can do. I can't bear the thought of wasting so much time. There's so much I want to do. Do you know anyone who might hire me—maybe part time?"

"I'll think about it. We should wait until we know more about your schedule."

"There's something else I need, Mom. Can you find a spiritual-type person I can talk to—like a spiritual counselor?"

"You know more ministers and priests than I do. What about someone from our church, or maybe one of the priests at Spring Hill College? Any of them would be glad to talk to you."

"That's not what I mean. I'm talking about an ordinary person,

maybe one of your friends you know can be trusted. I need someone I can just talk to about spiritual things. I don't want to be lec-
tured or preached to."

I thought of friends whom I had come to think of as spiritual
giants but couldn't picture myself asking them to take on such a
heavy responsibility.

"Let me think about that, too. We'll find the right person for
you."

Ross's schedule called for chemotherapy to begin on July 5th,
six days away. His friends called and visited often and his mail
basket soon filled. Two carloads of friends from Birmingham
came to visit and some of them were still around late Sunday
afternoon when plans had to be discussed for the trip to NIH.

I walked to the front yard where they were gathered and told
Ross I would like to go with him to NIH the next day.

"Mom, how many times do we have go through this? I've told
you a hundred times. I'm not a kid. I know what to expect from
the treatment. It's not necessary for you to go."

"It may not be necessary for you but maybe it is for me. I want
to know about these new drugs and how they affect you. Once
you get under way, I'll come home. I want to see first hand. After
that, you're on your own."

He rolled his eyes upward and shook his head. He turned to
his friends, looking for support. They glanced at me, then looked
away and said nothing.

"You sure do ask for punishment, Mom. You know I'd rather
handle this by myself. Why don't you let me do it my own way?"

"Please, Ross. Just this once. I think someone should be with
you. I promise not to hang around if you don't need me."

"Do you mean it? Will you promise to keep out of my room if
I don't need you?"

"Of course."

"Will you promise to let me handle my own affairs, including
this?"

"I promise."

"All right, then. But you have to come home when I tell you."

We visited a nearby shop which specialized in camping and
outdoor gear and purchased the large backpack he had selected

months before in preparation for his trip with Rebecca and James. Even with his crutches, he thought he could manage his own things for trips to NIH. After he finished with whatever awaited him, he still planned to travel.

When we arrived at NIH, we learned that his schedule called for an MRI at 8:00 a.m. the next day, to be followed by insertion of a neckline catheter to be used for all drawing of blood for tests, and for chemotherapy.

He had to go to surgery for the neckline catheter and was still groggy when he was returned to his room. I read the protocol sheet I had been given, the "road map" which outlined the order of treatment, but I wasn't asked to sign a consent form which listed the side effects. Ross no longer needed a parental co-signer. Ifosfamide was to be given first, followed by Etoposide (VP 16). Mesna was to be given periodically for 18 hours after each daily dosage. The drugs were to be given five days in a row, every three weeks. There would be 12 cycles given.

It was July 5, 1988. As I stood at the window looking at the skyline of Bethesda, I calculated that if all went well and there were no delays other than for the surgery, it could be finished in about one year.

When Ross was originally diagnosed in September, 1982, the shock of the word "cancer" and the amputation of his arm were comparable to an earthquake that shook our foundations and dropped us into a deep, black hole. The chemotherapy at that time was like a dark, slippery, perilous cave that had to be maneuvered very cautiously. We felt our way along each step. The current prospect of chemotherapy, then surgery, then chemotherapy again, triggered a scene of Ross standing at the foot of a steep, tall mountain with dark clouds swirling around sharp, jagged peaks.

There were no high hills to be seen from the hospital window in Bethesda, but Ross's mountain and its height were clearly before him. Many peaks, valleys, and plateaus were hidden by the ominous, perilous, whirling clouds. The mountain had to be scaled. And Ross had to travel alone. In my fantasy, I saw him as a gazelle—his head held high and his brown eyes alert and shining as he swiftly and gracefully moved from peak to peak.

He began his first step. Sedation and antiemetic drugs kept him very still and quiet through the first administering. When he awoke, he seemed disoriented and said he was nauseated. I prepared an emesis basin, stood by his bed, and waited. It wasn't needed. After several hours of sitting by his bedside, I left him and returned to the hotel.

The next morning when I arrived in his room, he asked me to pull the curtain around the bed and sit with him. He asked for ice water. His eyes were closed, with tears puddled in the corners. I straightened up his tray and table and noticed his wastebasket was full of used tissues. He was quiet all day.

Again, late in the afternoon, the drugs were given. More than two hours passed before both bottles were emptied. Again, the tears silently slipped down his cheeks.

This was the time I had planned to return to Mobile. It was true—he didn't need me for assistance when nauseated. The antiemetic drugs controlled the vomiting and his right arm was free because of the neckline catheter. With a pan prepared for sponge bathing, he could manage. But he was weak and dizzy. In order for him to go to the bathroom, he had to put on his prosthesis so he could use the crutches.

I went outside the building to think about what I should do. It seemed cruel to turn and walk away when he appeared so despondent. Although I had promised, I didn't think I could do it. He had three more days of the drugs coming up—that night, Friday and Saturday nights.

As I sat in front of the building pondering, I noticed there were larger crowds of people outside at this time. Two young men walked over and sat beside me. Handsome, strong, and healthy-looking in their bright-colored summer shorts and madras shirts, one of them asked where I was from.

When I told him, he said, "We live in California and we're trying to decide if we want to participate in AIDS research."

"Are you going to do it?" I asked.

"I don't think so. I doubt it. They want to inject us with a virus with symptoms similar to AIDS. It sounds risky and I'm afraid I'd lose my job."

"How did you hear about this?" I asked.

"An ad in *USA Today*. There are people here from all over the country. It's a good deal. Even if you don't want to participate, you still get a free trip to Washington and your hotel paid."

By 1988, AIDS had become a national issue, and we felt its significance on the pediatric floor of NIH as well. Once when I entered Ross's room, he asked if I had seen the demonstration in front of the Clinic Center. When I told him I hadn't, he said that the network news showed hundreds of protestors demanding that other research be suspended in favor of AIDS study and treatment.

From 1983, I recalled a roommate who was placed in the room with Ross one night after midnight. The young man had been brought by ambulance from a hospital in Baltimore. Ross was sedated, and, as he slept, the nervous and restless roommate wanted to talk. A handsome young man with dark, curly hair, his eyes widened as he lay in the bed with the covers pulled up to his chin. In whispered words, he told me that he had no idea what was wrong with him and didn't understand the emergency surrounding his condition. He explained that he had recently been in an exercise program when, rather suddenly, his stomach started getting larger and larger.

With so many different roommates and so many varying symptoms, I didn't attach any significance to his story until the next day. As I gathered Ross's things to get ready for discharge, I started to pick up the roommate's clothes from the bathroom floor when a nurse came in and said, "Leave those alone. Don't touch them."

Later, Ross wanted to take a shower before leaving the hospital and the nurse insisted he wait until he reached the hotel. In the hall, I noticed several impromptu gatherings of nurses in whispered conversations.

Before we left the room, a nurse who had been assigned to both the new roommate and Ross came in to talk to the young man. First, she apologized to him for not checking on him more often and explained that they had been instructed to keep out of the room unless it was necessary. Then she said, "When Ross is discharged, we're turning this room into an isolation unit and you'll be quarantined for a few days until we know more about your condition."

It slowly began to dawn on me. The emergency and need for isolation must have been because of AIDS. I wondered if anyone had considered Ross. In 1983, I had just heard of the condition, and thought that it hadn't been firmly established just exactly how it was transmitted.

At that time, there were no special sterile techniques in place on the pediatric floor for anything out of the ordinary except in the "flow room," where patients were placed after huge doses of chemotherapy combined with extensive radiation. Later, procedures were instituted for isolation and quarantine of AIDS patients, but they were soon discarded and all patients were treated the same.

In 1988, AIDS patients were on all floors of the hospital where they were being treated for whatever their condition required. I didn't know what was going on in the labs.

One of the things I noticed when entering Ross's room was a sturdy, red plastic box sitting on a table. Each patient's room had one. All used needles were dropped through a slit in the top, and I knew this was to protect the janitors from coming in contact with body fluids.

Also, outside the door in the hall, a box containing plastic gloves was fastened to the wall. They weren't sterile for patient protection, but were used to protect the nurses and other technicians.

There must have been sterile procedures in place to protect the patients from each other, but I never saw them, and nothing was ever said. They bathed in the same shower, shaved, and brushed their teeth in the same lavatory. I couldn't worry about it, though. At the moment, Ross had enough to deal with.

When the neckline catheter was put in place, Ross was told the tubes would have to be changed in three days in order to guard against infection. On Friday, that was done at 9:00 a.m. The large dressing over the point of entry had been changed daily by the hall nurse.

Before the drugs were started on Friday night, I walked over near Ross's bed and asked, "Are you awake?"

"Partly."

"I'm keeping my promise to you. I plan to go home tomorrow. Is that okay?"

"You don't have to leave if you don't want to," he mumbled. "I don't care if you want to stay. I hate to see you spend so much money on hotels."

"Don't worry about it. I'm in Rockville and it's not that expensive. I ride the shuttle to NIH. Don't look for something to worry about. Let's see how you do tonight."

"My neck is hurting."

"Where?"

"At the catheter."

"How long has it been hurting?"

"I don't know. Not long—just this afternoon."

"Have you told the nurse?"

"She looked at it but said everything was in place."

"Maybe you're just hurting all over. Does the chemo make you feel uncomfortable when it's going in?"

"I don't know. I'm so zonked out, I don't feel anything."

"Isn't it better to be zonked than sick?"

"I guess."

Ifosfamide and VP 16 were brought in. After the bottles were empty, he squirmed around in his bed trying to get comfortable. He complained again of his neck hurting. I concluded that, when they changed the tubes that morning, something must have caused an irritation.

The next morning, I checked out of the hotel and carried my luggage to the hospital. I made my plane reservation for Saturday night. When I went into Ross's room, he seemed terribly sick and was moaning about his neck hurting. He was shivering, so I went to the linen closet for blankets. I called for his nurse.

She checked and found he had a fever. As he began to shake

with chills, she quickly pulled the bandage from the catheter site and found a big glob of pus surrounding the incision.

She rushed out to find the hall doctor. Shortly after he came into the room and examined the site, a surgeon was summoned to place an IV in Ross's arm. Antibiotic was immediately started.

The Infectious Disease staff filed in and there was much flurry of activity. A nursing supervisor came up from the surgery department and brought his record. They seemed astonished and disbelieving that this could have happened.

Cultures were rushed to the lab. It would take several days to determine exactly what type of infection it was. The neckline catheter was removed. Preliminary diagnosis: staph infection, directly into his bloodstream.

Ten days from the start of the chemotherapy, Ross would have no ability to fight infection. This was the fourth day and his blood counts would start dropping in a day or two. It was a race against time to stem the spread of the infection before the white blood count started dropping.

I canceled my plane reservation. Mary came immediately when I called her. We took turns sitting by his bed all day and night.

Monday morning, he seemed to be improving. His fever was not quite so high and he said he felt better and was hungry.

"You gave us a scare, Ross," I said.

"I gave me one, too," he said. "I think I'm going to be okay now, if you want to think about going home."

"I'll think about it, but I'm not promising. Let's see how you do today."

The surgery department had sent someone in who managed to find a vein in his arm to insert the IV. This meant he couldn't get out of bed, since his right arm was strapped to a board and he was unable to use his crutches.

"Doesn't look like I'll be going anywhere for awhile," he said. "I think you can leave."

The next morning, I kissed him good-bye and caught the shuttle to the airport, not knowing if it was the right thing to do. It was important to me to stay, but I knew it was important to him that I go. And I had promised.

He stayed in bed for a week longer, getting the antibiotic. His white blood counts started dropping on Tuesday and reached bottom on Thursday.

Mary and Frank brought him special dinners from restaurants. Allan Riorda, his New Orleans cousin who now lived in Baltimore, brought his fiancee Melissa for a visit. Ross had telephone calls from friends who were scattered all over the United States—even some from Honduras and Japan. I spoke with him almost every day.

On Tuesday, he was dismissed from the hospital but had to stay in the area. I planned to return to Maryland but Mary assured me she could take care of him for a couple of days.

I said, "Mary, let me warn you. It's a big hassle getting out of the hospital."

"You worry too much, Mom. I can handle it."

"Just prepare yourself, and plan to be patient. Tell the nurse you need two wheelchairs and ask her if you can take one of them home with you. She knows you'll bring it back."

"Oh, Mom, it can't be that bad. I won't have any problems," she asserted.

Since it is a two-hour round trip from where she lived, I waited until evening to call her.

"Mom, it was the most ridiculous thing I've ever heard, trying to get out of that hospital! I've never in my whole life had such a frustrating experience. You wouldn't believe what I had to go through. And there was nobody to help me. I thought the elevator would never come. And when we finally got out, we hit the rush hour on the beltway and were stalled for another hour."

She had to take him back the next morning to the out-patient clinic for blood work. That night, he had chest pains and, when he checked his temperature, he found it was more than 100 degrees. He waited until daylight before he told Mary, "Let's go. I've got to go back."

She loaded most all his things into the car and drove back to the hospital. He was admitted with his fever rising and his chest hurting. Another neckline catheter was put in place and antibiotics were re-started. X-rays showed nothing in his lungs that could be causing the problems, but the pains continued through Friday night.

While he was still in the hospital, most of his hair came out. Mary got him on the plane on Monday and he arrived home— three weeks from the day he had left. He was in the hospital all but two days of that period.

When he visited Dr. Clarkson on Tuesday, I insisted on going with him in order to ask the same questions I had asked the doctors at NIH.

Dr. Clarkson had moved his office from the small cottage by Lyons Park to a sprawling modern complex attached to the Mobile Infirmary. Somehow, he looked much older than I remembered, and I wondered if he was overworking. I was comforted with his up-to-the-minute knowledge of cancer treatment.

"No, Ross, I don't think it's a metastasis," he said. Unfortunately, or fortunately, there's just not enough osteosarcoma to make a long-range study. If this was breast cancer we were talking about, I could quote statistics all day. Occasionally, when a woman has cancer in one breast and a mastectomy is done, she will develop another tumor in the other breast. The second tumor is not a metastasis. It's a separate, unrelated tumor. I can't be positive about bone cancer because we don't have enough evidence to study, but I personally don't believe it's a metastasis."

"I just wanted to let you know what's going on, Dr. Clarkson, in case I might need to call you," Ross said.

"Sure, Ross, I'll be glad to follow you like I did before. Make certain I know every time you come home, even if you don't need me. I want to let my partners know so they can be aware."

Ross took out the old brown suede hat and went to a hairdresser who shaved his head. We washed and repacked his clothes in the backpack. I tried to discourage him from taking so many things, but I failed. He took all the *Foreign Affairs* journals, some of his old college textbooks, a small tape player with earphones and several of his Windom Hill tapes.

In the evening, we searched the stores for a straw hat like the one a girlfriend had brought him from Mexico in the summer of 1983. The hat wasn't particularly unusual, but it had a jaunty look with a bright red headband. It was in tatters now, but nothing we saw in the stores could compare with it and we couldn't find anything else which satisfied him.

"Mom, help me figure out what I can wear on my head. It's too hot to wear this old suede thing, and besides, I have to take it off when I go inside. I want something I can leave on indoors, even when I'm in bed."

I didn't remind him of the Arab headdress he used before. I went upstairs and checked all my scarves and found a beautiful Italian silk which Mary had given to me. It was fine silk—dark mottled brown with a black edge. I took it downstairs.

"Sit down, Ross. Let's try something."

"What's that?"

"Just wait a minute. I said we're only going to try it."

"Is that a lady's scarf?"

"As a matter of fact, it's not. Someone gave it to Frank Lambert. He gave it to Mary, and she passed it on to me. So it's a man's scarf. And it's also very expensive."

"How expensive?"

"I would guess at least two hundred dollars—maybe more."

"That's ridiculous! No scarf can cost that much."

I fashioned the scarf, pirate-style, around his bald head and said, "Go look at yourself."

He went to the mirror and stood, turning his head from side to side.

"What do you think?" I asked.

"I like it okay. It feels real good. Do you think it looks stupid?"

"No, I think it looks spiffy. It's a handsome scarf."

"You know I can't tie it myself. You'll have to tie it for me. Can I have it?"

"It's yours if you want it."

"Now all I need is a patch over my eye and I'll look like a pirate."

Bill came in just as Ross was leaving and said, "You're not going out with that thing tied around your head, are you?"

"Yes, I am. I like it."

"Why don't you wear one of those mesh baseball caps with a visor like all the other patients up there?"

"Because I don't like caps. It's too hot to wear my hat, and I'm me. I'm not 'all the other patients up there'."

∽

Ross didn't object to me going with him on the trip to NIH the next day for round number two of chemotherapy because the first thing on the schedule, after a CT scan and before the start of treatment, was the implantation of a device in his chest to be used for all future chemotherapy, drawing of blood, or anything else requiring a needle. The Port-A-Cath, with good luck, would remain in place until he finished the protocol and he wouldn't have to be stuck again except for one single puncture through his skin into the device. Implanting the Port-A-Cath, though a common procedure, was surgery. He was scheduled for 8:00 Friday morning.

Mary dropped by the hospital after work Thursday evening. As we sat in Ross's room and talked, he said, "Mom, you don't have to rush over here in the morning. Why don't you just wait until about ten o'clock? I should be finished by then. Try to enjoy yourself a little. Drink your coffee and read the *Post*. And please bring me the *Post* when you finish with it."

"We'll see, Ross. I'll wait until I wake up to make that decision," I said, kissing him goodnight.

"See you in the morning," he said. "But don't hurry."

Early the next morning, I tried to think of ways to kill time until 10:00. I tried to follow Ross's instructions to drink coffee and read the paper. I showered and was getting dressed when, a few minutes after 7:00, the phone rang.

"Mom, could you come on over?"

"What's wrong, Ross?"

He cleared his throat and swallowed hard. "Nothing's happened yet. I just want you to come on over as soon as you can. I'll tell you about it when you get here."

"You're upset, aren't you?"

"I'm scared."

"I'm on my way. Be there in a few minutes."

When I rushed into his room, he looked at me with eyes wide and reddened and said, "He told me he might puncture my lung."

"Somebody's got a lot of nerve. Who said that?"

Between sniffling and taking deep breaths, he said that an anesthesiologist had been in to see him at 7:00 a.m. and matter-of-factly recited the routine statistics of all the problems that can happen when putting a Port-A-Cath in place. Puncturing the lung was one of them. Less than an hour before he was to be taken to surgery, he had to hear this gloomy possibility for the first time. I was fed up with brutal honesty.

"It's the lawyers," I said.

"What do you mean?"

"The medical profession, too. As long as a patient knows in advance of possible errors, the doctor will be held blameless."

"What are you talking about?"

"You shouldn't expect this is going to happen. The doctor is just trying to protect himself from a lawsuit."

He turned his head on the pillow and gazed out the window.

"If he did puncture your lung and you tried to sue him, he could always say that you knew the risks."

"It wouldn't hold up in court."

"It probably would," I said.

The more we thought about the absurdity of the concept, the funnier it became. We fabricated courtroom scenes where imaginary surgical snafus were being presented to the jury.

When the orderlies arrived and got him settled on the gurney to start moving into the hall, he had a weak smile and a "thumbs-up" sign.

I walked with him to the surgery door and kissed him on the forehead. When the big double doors closed, I sat on a nearby bench, breathed deeply, and counted to ten. Was it really necessary to scare a patient half to death just before wheeling him to the operating room?

After getting a cup of coffee in the cafeteria, I went back to the bench near the door. Soon, an attendant propped the door open as Ross was being rolled along the hall on a gurney. Attractive nurses walked on each side of him. The bed was raised and Ross sat upright, smiling and chatting with the girls. I wished I could be invisible and fade out of the scene, because I knew he would have preferred that his mother not be there.

From surgery, he was taken to the 13th floor, the pediatric wing. The hall seemed quieter than I remembered, yet there were more rooms than there had been on the sixth floor in 1982. Each door had two patients' names on it, so I knew the hall was filled.

Ross's room had more space than I recalled from the sixth floor. It looked clean and bright. Happy, primitive oil paintings—early American scenes depicting home and family—faced each patient's bed. A small television on a retractable arm was within reach of the patient. The ceiling had a unique lighted design of white fluffy clouds slowly moving in a blue sky.

A space for a caregiver had been added. A narrow bunk-type bed, built into the wall at the foot of each patient's bed, had a thin, opaque curtain to hide the sleeper from the traffic. Under this bed were cabinets for storing luggage. Once Ross was settled in his bed, I went back to my hotel, got my things and checked out. I now had my own space at the hospital, and again claimed the title of "caregiver."

A laundry room and bathroom with shower at the end of the hall contributed to the home-away-from-home. The family room had a stove, microwave oven, toaster, refrigerator—and, of course, the inescapable television set which blared constantly. There was a telephone watts line for our use at certain hours of the day and evening. Crafts were available, and the library sent a cart of books down every day. The short-order line in the cafeteria in the basement remained open 24 hours a day. All that was missing was a friend from home.

Neither one of the two chemotherapy drugs nor the follow-up drug, mesna, was expected to cause any problems with the kidneys. Yet, already, the magnesium problems of the past recurred. His kidneys failed to filter properly, causing loss of magnesium, which was manifest in severe cramps throughout his body. Again, a daily handful of tablets was prescribed.

Ifosfamide and VP 16 were begun that night through the newly implanted Port-A-Cath. Ross didn't complain about the needle. He had to be carefully watched now for signs that his body was trying to reject the device. At least his lung wasn't punctured.

Again, the antiemetic drugs seemed to play havoc with his emotions and by the third day, he couldn't stop the tears from silently sliding down his face. Nurses tried to offer words of encouragement. Often, during the night, I could see the light from the hall as the door was being opened and I could hear the nurse whisper, "What do you need, Ross?"

"Are you busy?" he asked.

"Sort of. You need something?"

"Can you sit with me and talk?"

"I'll be back as soon as I can."

There could not have been much time to spend just talking. Many very young patients were in the pediatric wing at this time. A crying baby, about three months old, whimpered on its father shoulder as the young man walked back and forth along the hall, patting the child on its back.

One day, when in the family room, I asked another mother, "Do you know what's wrong with the little baby?"

"AIDS," she said. "There are several small children on the hall with AIDS."

"What about the mother? Where is she?"

"I think she's in treatment, too. The father was a drug user and infected the mother before the baby was born."

While we were talking, a little girl about three years old came into the family room, followed by an older lady who was pushing the child's IV pole. "Watch out for the table...don't run into the chair. Go real slow," the lady said. The child had a bandage over her eye, and, as they left the room, the lady continued to warn her of things in her path.

"Do you know anything about that little girl?" I asked.

"Another case of AIDS. The child is going blind and has had one eye removed. That's the grandmother with her."

"What about the parents?"

"Who knows? The mother dumped the kid with her parents when she found out it had AIDS."

Over the years, I had heard of several fathers who had left home when a child was diagnosed with a catastrophic problem, but this was my first knowledge of the mother of a patient on the pediatric wing of the Clinic Center who had left her suffering child.

26

August, 1988

As soon as Ross was able to travel, we returned home. He was quite ill, and, although he had taken only two cycles of chemo, he was already losing weight. His appetite was slow in returning. Nothing tasted like he expected.

He visited Dr. Clarkson's office three times that week to get blood work done. During the following week, he announced that he was going to Montgomery and Birmingham for the weekend to visit college friends. His white blood count was very low.

"Here we go again, Ross. I can't tell you what to do. You know the risks of infection."

"I can go into a hospital in Montgomery or Birmingham just as easily as the Mobile Infirmary if I have to."

"Sure, just drive up to the emergency room and say, 'Give me a couple of gallons of antibiotic please—and put it through my Port-A-Cath.' Simple as that, huh?"

"I told Dr. Clarkson I was going. He said if I had any problem to call him and he would get in touch with someone in either place," he said. "Let's get this straight right now: I'm not going to sit around the house and wait to die. I'm going to live while I can."

"Go for it," I said, wishing I could live that well.

"And while I'm gone, try to think of someone I can talk with about spiritual things. I want to see somebody before I have to go back to NIH."

The next day, after Ross left, I had a phone call from a man I had met recently. A mutual friend had told him about Ross, and he wanted to express his interest and concern.

He was a vice-president of a local bank, a deacon in the Catholic church, and had led seminars and taught religion classes at Spring Hill College. He invited me to lunch that day.

Paul Sheldon came to my office and drove us to a nearby cafe. A handsome, gentle man with intense blue eyes and a quick smile, he spoke to several friends as he held my arm and ushered me to a table in the back corner of the restaurant.

Since we didn't know each other very well, he began by telling me a little about himself. He felt his true calling was in counseling and ministering to people in need. He spoke of his family—his wife, Jennie, and their four children. Although he didn't verbalize sympathy, I could tell he had compassion.

We parried a little about my family and Ross in particular. "Not here—not now," I said. "I'm sorry. I can't talk about it. But thanks for being willing to listen. I'll keep it in mind."

"Promise me one thing," he said as he reached across the table and took my hand. "Do something for yourself. You'll be no good for Ross if you don't take care of you. You can't shoulder this alone and you don't have to. Turn to a friend. Don't keep it bottled in. Do something good for yourself. Promise?"

Looking down into my cup of coffee, I nodded my head. "Okay...I'll try," I said.

On Saturday morning, I thought about what Paul had said: "Do something for yourself." I called my sister Dorothy in New Orleans and told her I would like to drive over to spend the night. She encouraged me to come.

As I was putting some things in my overnight bag, I thought of Paul again, and suddenly it dawned on me. Here was Ross's spiritual counselor. I called him and told him I was taking his advice by planning to drive to New Orleans and listen to my favorite tapes while on the interstate. I asked if he would consider taking the responsibility of being a spiritual counselor to Ross.

He admitted that he had never counseled anyone who had been through what Ross had, or one who was facing what he had to face, but he was willing to try.

As I drove along the highway on a beautiful Saturday morning, I realized that a burden had been lifted from me. Paul, like many others before him, had appeared when he was needed. I thought of others who had come into Ross's life unexpectedly and when needed most. My prayers for him were being answered without my praying, and all there was left for me to do was say, "Thank you."

From many years ago, I remembered a book I had read by a lady named Corrie ten Boom. The name of the book was *The Hiding Place*. I had long ago forgotten the details of the story, but remembered that Corrie ten Boom was a Christian Dutch lady who was imprisoned for hiding Jews in her home at the time of the holocaust during World War II. What I recalled from her story was that we should be thankful for all things, in all situations—not just the good things. Be thankful—no matter how bad things appeared. A man named Paul had first said the same thing 2,000 years ago as recorded in the scriptures.

I could see nothing to be thankful for in Ross's situation. But, according to my memory of *The Hiding Place*, we were to be thankful, period. Somewhat like unconditional love. Be thankful in *all* things.

I had always assumed that I had to recognize a blessing in order to be thankful for it. It was beginning to faintly dawn on me that maybe this wasn't the right way at all. Hanging on to this thread of a thought, I didn't know if I could do it but was ready to give it a try.

With resolve, I made up my mind that my private motto was going to be: Have a Grateful Heart, no matter how bleak the situation appeared, or more accurately, *in spite of*.

At first, the idea seemed defiant, but I learned that it was also energizing. I was determined to have a grateful heart, no matter what. But I didn't know where to begin.

However, I made a remarkable discovery. There was no room within me for sadness, fear, self-pity, anger, guilt or any other destructive emotion, when I could achieve the grateful heart. If only I could learn to maintain it.

∾

When Ross returned from Birmingham, I told him that I had found someone for him to talk with about spiritual things.

"You found somebody? Who is it?"

"Paul Sheldon."

"Who's he?"

"A man I know. I asked him and he said he would like to meet you."

"Great! Do you think he could see me tomorrow?"

Paul gave Ross an appointment on Wednesday and he went downtown to his office for the meeting.

When I arrived home from work, I asked, "How was it? How did it go?"

"Good. He's a real nice guy. I think I could talk to him about most anything. He didn't preach at me. I'm to call him when I get back from NIH."

We packed his bag and he left the next day for Maryland for the third round of chemotherapy. This time he went alone.

∾

Before the treatment began, I telephoned his room. A man named Daullary answered, and I realized Ross had a roommate I hadn't met. Mr. Daullary sounded very upset, but courteously said he would tell Ross that I had called. Later, when Ross returned my call, I asked about his roommate.

"His name is Mark and he's just a kid. He's very sick."

"What's wrong with him?"

"Leukemia. He's been in remission for a couple of years and just recently relapsed. His mom and dad are real upset."

"Can you call me when you feel like going down to the watts line? I don't want to ring the room again."

"I'm okay, Mom, and I'm not going to promise I'll call. I may not feel like getting out of bed and waiting in line to use the phone. Don't worry about me. If I need anything, I'll call you, and if you don't hear from me, you'll know I'm okay."

He didn't call back, but on Wednesday, when I called the nurses' station, I found that he was out on a pass.

"Out on a pass? You're kidding! Doesn't he have a treatment tonight?" I asked.

"He'll be back in time for treatment. He's gone to Camp Fantastic—one of the social workers took him."

"But doesn't he have a dose of mesna this afternoon?"

"He'll get it. He has a backpack with a portable pump."

"Isn't he nauseated and dopey?"

"He's a little sleepy and nauseated, but he wanted to go and Donna Geller volunteered to take him."

Ross was right. He didn't need me and was doing much better without me.

Bill and I met him at the arrival gate when he came home. Wearing his pirate scarf, he slowly hobbled up the ramp on his crutches. He looked so thin and frail. But he had a smile on his face for having gone through this round of treatment alone. After the many, many sessions with chemotherapy, it was a first.

Early in the following week, we began to plan the clothes he would need for the extended stay in Maryland following the surgery.

Ross met with Paul Sheldon again. Ross had recently been given a small bottle of holy water by Catholic friends, and had no idea how to use it. He asked Paul to talk with him about it and explain its significance. That conversation led Paul to arrange a healing service.

Paul requested permission from the priests at Spring Hill College to conduct the service on campus. He also asked Father Bobby Rimes to assist.

On Labor Day, Paul and his wife Jennie, several priests, about fifteen of Ross's college friends, along with Ross, Bill and I, gathered in the student chapel.

The rite of anointing with oil was done by the priests and Paul, who was now wearing a clerical collar. Then, Bill and I were asked to stand behind Ross with our hands on his shoulder. Everyone else was asked to place a hand on Ross, Bill, or me. Father Rimes prayed, asking God for Ross's healing, ending with all of us praying the Lord's Prayer. Ross sat quietly in the middle of the group, and, at the "amen," he hugged everyone.

Early the next morning, he left for Maryland, riding with a former Spring Hill College student, Dave Joudis, who was returning to his home in North Carolina. He offered to drive Ross on to Maryland.

27

September, 1988

CAT scans were scheduled again on Friday, and after Ross was finished, he was sent to George Washington University Hospital for a bone scan. Either there was something wrong with NIH's equipment, or they were short-staffed—I never knew why he was sent to GWU.

Since he was so near Capitol Hill when he finished the bone scan, he paid a call on Congressman Callahan's office. The staff arranged an impromptu party, and everyone went out to dinner at Julio's. Someone drove him all the way to Bethesda—back to the Marriott.

Surgery was scheduled for Thursday, and I flew up to Washington on Sunday. At Dr. Malawer's request, Ross again went to Children's Hospital for another angiogram on Monday. We were there from 8:30 a.m. until 6:00 p.m. When he finally got back to NIH and went through the admissions process, it was 7:00 p.m. before we reached the 13th floor.

A nurse looked up and, with hands on her hips, said, "Well, well—look who finally decided to come to the hospital."

"What do you mean?" Ross asked.

"Where in the world have you been, Ross? We've been looking all over for you. We've been expecting you all day."

"Why? Didn't you know I was at Children's Hospital?"

"No one told us. And where were you Friday? The clinic was looking everywhere for you. They called here several times."

"What did they want? They're the ones who sent me to George Washington for a bone scan."

"They tried to call you there and you were already gone. But you didn't come back."

"I didn't know I was supposed to. It was after four o'clock when I finished at GWU and the Clinic closes at four. What did they want?"

"You'd better find your doctor and ask him."

Dr. Malcolm Smith, Ross's Clinical Associate, had floor duty that night. He met us in the hall.

Slightly built, his long white hospital coat seemed too big. He peered at us through large, black horn-rimmed glasses, and spoke in a soft, southern drawl. He shifted from one foot to the other before saying, "Ross, your CT scan last Friday showed a suspicious spot in your lung. It appears to be a nodule."

Ross looked at me, then quickly looked away. He turned his back to the doctor and lifted his eyes to the ceiling.

"It's very tiny, Ross, but we compared other scans and it wasn't there before."

Ross clenched my hand. After a few seconds of silence, he turned around to face the doctor and asked, "What happens now? Will the surgery go on as scheduled?"

"I'm almost certain it will, Ross, but we have to do more tests. We're going to repeat the CT of your chest tomorrow."

Ross took a few steps along the hall away from us. I stood silently, rubbing my brow while staring at the floor.

"Try not to worry, Mrs. Phelps," Dr. Smith said. "It could be a number of things. We have to take a closer look and watch it carefully."

Ross sauntered back towards us, took a deep breath, and said, "Go on to the hotel, Mom. I'm okay."

"I can stick around for awhile. I'm in no hurry."

"It's not necessary. I'm all right."

I returned to the hotel and tried to pray. Remembering my

resolve to keep a grateful heart, I tried to be thankful for CT scans and X-rays.

He was given a battery of tests and scans for the next two days and conferences were held. On Wednesday, we were told that surgery would be performed on his lungs as soon as he recuperated from the surgery on his leg. The limb-sparing procedure would go on as scheduled.

∾

The staff of nurses and social workers began to pay closer attention to Ross and were often in his room, encouraging him to discuss his feelings. A nurse told him about a popular book she had been reading.

Ross asked me, "Have you ever heard of Dr. Bernie Siegel?"

"Yes, I bought one of his books a year ago, *Love, Medicine and Miracles*. Why?"

"One of the nurses told me I should read it."

"You were so busy with school I didn't think you had time to get into it." And you weren't thinking about cancer, I didn't add.

"Did you bring it with you?"

"No, I gave it to a friend whose husband had cancer. I told her she could keep it."

"Do you think you could get me a copy? What's it about? Should I read it?"

"I don't know—I have mixed feelings about it. A lot of the things Dr. Siegel has to say aren't new to me or you, but you'd have to read it for yourself."

The shops in the basement of the Clinic Center did not have a copy, and I wondered why. However, I found one in Bethesda, and also picked up a copy of *Getting Well Again*, written by a husband and wife team, Doctors Carl and Stephanie Simonton, with James L. Creighton. Carl Simonton was an oncologist, and Stephanie Simonton a psychologist.

Dr. Siegel is a surgeon at Yale, and the Simontons, at the time their book was written, were in Texas. Their work was similar and related. At last, attention was being paid to the physical effects of mental attitudes, especially as they related to the progression and treatment of cancer.

I knew that many members of the medical profession would reject these theories or anything else they didn't consider traditional medical practices. I recalled a conversation with Dr. Clarkson in Mobile more than five years before:

"Dr. Clarkson, I know you'll think I'm stupid, but can you tell me anything about laetrile?" I asked.

"Oh, no. Don't tell me that old remedy is rearing its head again. I thought it was finally dead and buried."

"I have to ask. Please be patient with me."

"All I can tell you is that it's been proven totally worthless in the treatment of cancer. There are some patients who still believe in it. You know, it's not available in this country, and there's no reason it should be. Ross is doing okay. Just forget about it."

"We'll try anything that might help—even if it's unproven. We'll go to Mexico to get the drug if we have to."

"Forget it, Mrs. Phelps. Let's stick with what we do know."

"All right. But don't be surprised if I call you back with more questions. I may even decide to take him to Lourdes."

"Why don't you take him to Paris instead? I think Ross would like Paris."

"Maybe we'll do that, too. I just want you to know that we'll go anywhere and try anything if we want to."

That conversation seemed eons away as I approached Dr. Smith in the hall later in the day. I asked him if he was familiar with Dr. Siegel's book.

"Oh yes, I've heard about it," he said in his usual kind voice. "I haven't read it and don't know of any clinical evidence available which has tested his theories."

"What do you think of it?"

"Based on what I've heard, I'm not for it. It seems to put the burden of getting well on the patient. I'm against that."

"Dr. Siegel doesn't recommend stopping treatment or refusing any available means of help. What I've read emphasizes that doctor's orders must be followed."

"Nevertheless, the patient is expected to hold certain attitudes, think certain thoughts, and believe in things they don't really understand. I think it's been proven that you can't meditate cancer into remission."

"I think Ross has been practicing similar attitudes for six years already. I don't see anything wrong with it."

"I didn't say there's anything wrong with it. It's just that I wouldn't want my patients to think they have to worry about whether they're following all the prescribed routines. I don't want them to feel they have failed if they have a relapse. That doesn't seem fair."

I hadn't thought of it that way, and agreed with his compassionate response. "How would you feel if Ross decided to practice this seriously?"

"I can't stop him, but I certainly don't recommend it. I want Ross to trust his drugs, trust us and the surgeons, and believe in what we're doing here."

"Really, Dr. Smith. Hasn't Ross already proven that he has trusted all those things since 1982? In view of these new developments, could you blame him for seeking other avenues for help? What else is there for him?"

"As I said, Mrs. Phelps, I can't stop him," he said, and slowly walked away.

Ross read Dr. Siegel's book. It hadn't been written in 1982, although similar ones had been available. At that time, the shock I was in would have prohibited concentration on anything, and Ross, being only 18 years old and in deep distress, would not have been open to a radically different way of thinking.

But now, as the hours moved closer and closer to the time for surgery, Ross found a small measure of peace and comfort in reading Dr. Siegel's book.

Surgery was to begin at 8:00 a.m. Thursday, September 15, 1988, two weeks short of exactly six years since his arm amputation.

The night before surgery, Ross got a pass from the hospital. Bill had arrived, so he and Mary joined us when we went to dinner at the Bello Mondo. Mary kept up her usual chatter, trying to distract Ross. She even had him laughing a few times.

Although Dr. Malawer had tried to explain to Ross and me a little about the surgery, it sounded so complicated that I gave up trying to understand thoroughly. When he told us of the amount of bone to be removed and that the knee would be replaced, my mind went blank, and not much else got through.

The prosthesis to be implanted was made of titanium and, if all went well and Ross took extreme precautions, it should last about 12 years. When that time came, no doubt there would be great advances in the field of limb-sparing surgery.

The muscles in his leg were to be re-positioned and the nerves and blood vessels would be re-routed accordingly. If all went well, over the years, bone might slowly re-grow over the metal implant.

The prosthesis should work well, with flexibility in the knee. Physical therapy was to begin soon after surgery, and Ross should be able to walk almost normally. He could never run again.

He could never jog, run to catch a train or plane, dash across a busy street, rush to shelter from a storm, play soccer, tennis, basketball or any sport which required running or jumping. No water or snow skiing or anything which could put extreme stress on his leg. There was always golf—if he had two hands. But he would be able to walk.

The extreme caution turned my thoughts to all the things he had enjoyed in the past—his reckless abandon as a goalie on the high school soccer team, running around the track, water skiing in the rivers and bays of Mobile and Baldwin Counties in Alabama, snow skiing in the Rockies and North Carolina, and the informal sessions of beach volleyball, touch football, and team-frisbee. He had keen agility and dexterity, a high energy level, and strong stamina. Although he didn't often have the opportunity to visit mountain slopes in the winter, he was an excellent snow skier. Since the amputation of his arm, he had hoped and planned to learn to ski without using poles.

He was seven years old at Christmastime in Aspen, Colorado, when he was introduced to the sport. We hadn't been able to find rental ski boots that would fit his and Scott's narrow feet, so while Bill and Mary were skiing, the two boys escaped from me, rode the T-bar up the "bunny" slope, and came flying down, jackets flapping, as they "skied" on their slick-soled Wellington boots.

On subsequent trips with friends or family, Ross became an excellent skier, traversing the highest slopes of the Rockies.

All this activity would be terminated for Ross, but I had to believe other techniques would be developed in the future. The knowledge and courage of Dr. Malawer and his colleagues amazed and humbled me.

The surgeons considered asking Ross to sign a consent for amputation of his leg in case anything went wrong during the operation, but Dr. Malawer decided against it. If anything was discovered that he didn't anticipate, he would stop the surgery and rethink the procedure.

When Mary, Bill, and I arrived at Ross's room at 7:00 a.m., it was full of people. I wondered if anyone had recited the litany of all the things that could go wrong.

Ross was limp and groggy when he was placed on the gurney. An elevator had been called and was waiting for him. All of us crowded into the car with his nurse and orderlies and rode to the surgery floor.

"Looks like you're going to a party, Ross," the elevator operator said to him. "All these folks your people?"

"Yes, my dad, my mom, and my sister," Ross said sleepily. "My brother couldn't come. He's taking care of the cats."

He was wheeled along the hall to the double doors. Mary walked close beside him and held his hand as Bill and I followed.

"Hugs and kisses time, Ross. This is as far as they can go," said his nurse.

We managed to keep our faces straight until we leaned over to kiss him. We lingered at the door and watched as the gurney moved far down the hall and turned a corner.

Mary left for work, Bill went for a long walk, and I strolled around on the grounds. As I sat on a bench under an oak tree, I shivered in the early fall breeze. Acorns fell around me and I picked some up and put them in my pocket. They were different from the acorns at home, and I wondered what species they were.

After wandering around the grounds for an hour, I returned to the surgery reception area. Bill soon arrived from his walk carrying newspapers.

"Any word?" he asked.

"No, it's too soon. Maybe it means 'so far, so good'."

"You know how long the surgery will take?"

"I didn't ask. I'm sure they don't know."

Dr. Malawer's statement that he would stop the surgery if he needed to remained on my mind. As the hours passed, I was thankful he didn't walk out with news that the surgery couldn't be done. I hadn't expected the calmness I felt, and wondered if people were praying for Ross and for the rest of us.

At 6:00 p.m., Dr. Malawer and Dr. Cook of the surgery staff came into the waiting room still dressed in their green scrub clothes. They didn't have much to say, but Dr. Malawer seemed pleased. It had gone well. Dr. Cook had assisted. They had been operating for 10 hours.

They told us Ross would be in the Intensive Care Unit through the weekend but we could probably see him for a few minutes later that night.

I telephoned Mary, then Scott, and my sister Vilma in Mobile and asked them to let others know. It was over and the doctors said it had gone well.

Mary returned to the hospital and joined us in our vigil. It was almost 10:00 p.m. before we were called to come in to the surgical ICU.

It seemed very dark in the huge room, with patients behind every curtain. We were led to Ross's space. Two nurses were with him, one intently watching the monitor at the foot of his bed, the other standing near his head.

Ross was writhing in agony, turning his head and moaning loudly. "Don't come in here!" he shouted. "I don't want you to see me. Please leave!" His entire body was shaking.

"He's been given morphine," said the nurse. "He doesn't know what he's saying."

Ross knew exactly what he was saying.

I said, "Ross, it's all over and Dr. Malawer is very pleased. Do you really want us to leave?"

"Yes. Please go!"

As Bill, Mary, and I walked along the hall, we could still hear his screams. We didn't talk when we were in the car. Mary drove us to our hotel then continued her long journey home.

None of us slept much that night. Mary confessed that she gave up trying to get to sleep, sat up in bed, and wrote a poem which she later shared with me:

> There is no Monday
>   or Friday or Saturday:
> just the neverending stream
>   of day and night,
> of day's beginning when
>   we are let in
> of night's signal when
>   we are sent out.
>
> And the only memories
>   we have of this time
> are times when we cried
>   or didn't cry enough
> or tying the thin thread
>   that was the continuity
> of our lives
>   with cars and traffic and highways
>
> of the Potomac from the north
>   and the Potomac from the south
>
> of things left undone
>   and things unimportant
> of the bare essentials
>   that define living
> and the essence of our existing
>   that is life.

28

Bill had become a serious and committed walker and decided to hike to the hospital the next morning. When we met later at the nurses' station, we asked them to call ICU and check on Ross.

"We have his bed ready," the nurse said. "He'll be up soon."

"No, he's not coming on the hall," I said. "He's to stay in ICU through the weekend."

"Plans must have been changed, Mrs. Phelps. He should be here by noon. It's the weekend and ICU may be understaffed."

Shortly after noon, he was brought in on a gurney. Lifting him to his bed required several people. He groaned loudly and constantly.

I apologized to his roommate, Tommy, and his mother, Beth. They assured me that I shouldn't worry. It couldn't be helped.

Nurses were constantly at Ross's side. Bill and I sat quietly at the foot of his bed and wrote notes to each other.

"Can you stay tonight?" I scribbled and passed the pad to Bill.

He handed it back to me. "I'll try. I'll have to go back to the hotel to get something to sleep in."

"Bring Ross's wool socks and his warm-up suit—they're in my bag." The note pad exchanged hands.

"O.K., anything else?"

I shook my head, trying to think what else might be needed.

"Have you had lunch?" I wrote.

He nodded his head, motioning his finger down, indicating the cafeteria.

"How was it?"

He passed the pad back to me. "Yuk!"

I scribbled on the note pad, "Could you bring me some candy bars? Go back to the hotel and rest. Come back tonight and I'll leave."

I don't think Ross was aware of where he was or that we were there. He begged for water and I tried to give him tiny bits of ice but he drifted back into the netherlands of morphine and pain before it reached his lips. He didn't stop moaning and turning his head, "Oh, Mom...oh, Mom...help me, help me!" Sometimes his eyes were open wide but they had a glassy look.

When Bill returned that night, I went to the hotel, and when I arrived back in the room the next morning, Bill looked haggard and exhausted. "I'm no good at this," he said. "Ross doesn't like my bedside manner."

"What do you mean? What happened?" I asked.

"Nothing happened. I couldn't do anything right. Nothing I did pleased him."

"Welcome to the club," I said. "Go on to the hotel and go to bed. We'll work out something for tonight."

Waves of pain engulfed Ross and he cried out again and again. A heavy cast was on his leg, yet he tried to turn his body, seeking a moment of relief.

On the other side of the curtain, Tommy struggled to get out of his bed, no doubt to get away from the noise and commotion. A tall, handsome young man with dark hair and moustache, Tommy appeared to be near Ross's age. When I asked, he said, "I'll be twenty years old tomorrow."

"What a coincidence. Tomorrow is Ross's twenty-fourth birthday."

Tommy was extremely limited in his ability to walk. Concern for him prompted me to ask the nurse if there was any other space available. She told me they were completely filled.

"It's not fair to the roommate," I said. "He seems to be very uncomfortable."

"Tommy's surgery on his hip was a long time ago. That's not what he's in the hospital for this time," she said.

All day and all night Saturday, Ross continued to call out for help and more pain medication. As I sat beside his bed, the moment my head began to nod, he would cry out. I expected the pain to be severe, but not this bad. His morphine gave only moments of relief and he suffered torturously.

Sunday morning, Bill checked out of the hotel and came to the hospital to say good-bye. He helped me put up birthday decorations I had brought from home and we had streamers and balloons all over the room for both boys. I tried to show Ross a new shirt I had bought for him, but he hardly noticed. Mary came in with brownies, which Frank's mother had sent in lieu of a birthday cake. The nurses brought ice cream and joined us in singing "Happy Birthday" to the two boys. It was a stupid thing for us to do. It was a miserable day for both of them.

Late in the afternoon, after Bill left, I saw Dr. Malawer in the hall, walking very fast toward Ross's room.

"Come with me," he ordered. "You can help me."

I was several steps behind him and I increased my pace to catch up, wondering how in the world he thought I could help him. I noticed that, although he had on a tweed sport coat, he wore blue jeans. The pleat in the back of his coat was opened wide because of a pair of garden shears in his back pocket. I assumed that he had been clipping hedges in his yard before coming to the hospital.

Dr. Malawer told me to stand on the other side of Ross's bed. Then he whisked the shears from his pocket and began to cut the cast away. It was a very long cast, from Ross's hip to the end of his toes. As Dr. Malawer cut from top to bottom, he asked me to hold the cast open. He never called for a nurse.

Finally reaching the end of the cast, he told me to place my hands under Ross's leg and slowly lift it while he moved the opened cast. When he slid the cast away, I gradually eased Ross's leg down onto the bed.

Ross didn't cry out, but he glared at me. I glared back.

Dr. Malawer removed the gauze and bandage from the surgery site. He said something about the cast being necessary to prevent swelling. The leg looked ghastly to me but I could tell Dr. Malawer was pleased with the surgery site.

I looked at Ross's foot. It had a black substance across the top, about four or five inches long from above his instep, almost to his toes, varying in width from a half inch to about two inches. Another black streak crossed the back of his heel. I wondered why they had painted something on his foot so far from the surgery site.

Dr. Malawer explained that Ross's leg swelled so badly during the operation, there wasn't enough skin to stretch across the surgery site. He had an eight-inch long, diamond-shaped area of raw, uncovered flesh.

In spite of the horror of it, there was no sign of excessive redness or infection. It looked clean and neat. The first skin grafts over the opened area were scheduled for the coming Friday. I didn't ask about the black areas on his foot.

Dr. Malawer called the nurses' station for bandages and he rewrapped the leg. When he asked for a brace, it was discovered there were none that would fit Ross. Physical Therapy was closed on Sunday.

"Find a brace," Dr. Malawer ordered the nurse.

He left the room with instructions to Ross to remain very still. As I walked toward the ice machine, I spotted him in an office, talking on the phone. I thought his face looked reddened, and he had wrinkles in his brow.

Finally, a brace was located, but it was far too large for Ross. It must have been designed for a taller, heavier person. But we had to make do—it was all that could be found. Pillows were brought in to elevate his leg so it would be higher than his heart.

On Monday, his brace was found and a gym bar was installed over his bed so he could reach up with his right hand and try to get more comfortable. The morphine continued. Still, he suffered endlessly. He cried for the pillows to be moved and adjusted all day and night, seemingly about every five minutes.

I don't know what I was thinking when I had asked Bill to bring socks and clothes for Ross. He had to remain stark naked under the sheets.

"Mom...you're going to have to help me...I can't bathe myself, you know," he breathlessly said.

"I'm going to help you. Tell me how you want to do it."

"Put water in a pan. Put a towel on the bed. Put the pan on it."

Talking drained him of energy he needed for resisting the pain. I placed the pan of water on the side of the bed.

"That's too cold. Put warm water in the pan."

I whirled back to the sink and added hot water.

"Now you've got it too hot! Get a bath cloth. Wet it...now put a tiny little bit of facial scrub on it."

"Facial scrub? A tiny little bit?"

"Come here and I'll show you...just a little squirt—a little circle—not too much. Sprinkle a little water on top of the scrub. Rub it in the bath cloth. Just a little. Not too much."

I handed him the prepared cloth and he vigorously scrubbed his face. "That's enough, Ross. Let's rinse your face."

"Change the water in the pan—and get the temperature right this time."

"There's nothing wrong with this water...."

"Just do as I ask, will you?" He looked as if he might burst into tears.

"Okay, okay, I'll change the water."

"Now, hand me my shampoo. Put some water on my head and a little bit of shampoo in my hand."

"Let's don't use shampoo. It'll be hard to rinse."

With a quivering chin, he said, "Don't tell me what to do. Give me some clean, wet bath cloths." He sloshed the cloth over his bald head. "Now, change the water. Get a clean bathcloth...wet it...soap it with Ivory—nothing else."

He was concentrating very hard to keep his plan working in the order he had rehearsed. Every few minutes, he leaned back on the pillow, closed his eyes, and breathed hard.

"You'll have to wash my arms and my back. Let me rest a minute. I can wash my chest and stomach. Go outside the curtain until I get through. Put some Dial soap on a bath cloth. Don't leave."

"I'm not going anywhere. I do need to go across the hall and get more bath cloths."

"See if you can find something besides paper cloths. Don't they have anything else in there?"

When I returned, he called, "You can come in now. I need you to change the water so I can rinse. Then I need you to help me finish."

I obeyed his orders, then turned back to the bed. "Okay. What next? How do we do this?"

"I'm going to lift myself up with the gym bar. I want you to finish washing my hips and my leg. Don't touch my right leg."

"I wouldn't dare touch your right leg."

"Go easy, Mom. You've got to work fast. I can't hold myself up for long. And don't move the sheet off me. Just reach under the sheet as soon as I can lift up. Ready?"

Blindly, I reached under the sheet. As he grasped the bar to lift himself, his arm shuddered, calling on all his strength.

"All finished, Ross. That's good enough. Let's quit for now."

"No. Change the water and the bath cloth. You have to rinse the soap off."

"Ross...."

"Please, please, do what I ask!"

"We need to change your sheets. They're all wet."

"Give me a few minutes. After you change the sheets, I want you to put lotion all over my body—just like we did the bath. I want to brush my teeth first. Let me rest a minute."

I prepared his toothbrush, a glass of water, and a basin.

"What kind of toothpaste is that?" he asked.

"I don't know. Whatever was in your hospital packet."

"You know I don't like that! Find my dopp kit and get my toothpaste. Wash all that other stuff out of my brush."

Like a robot, I followed his commands.

"Why do you put so much paste on the brush? That's too much. Please, please watch what you're doing!"

He propped himself up on the stump of his left arm and attacked his teeth with a vengeance. "Now, hand me a clean towel. Move all this stuff and change the sheets. Be careful with my leg...go easy when you lift it."

He grasped the bar again as I pulled away the wet sheet and

slipped the new one under him. After changing his six pillows, finally, we were finished—except for the rite of the lotions.

I asked, "Can we rest for a little while? We can do the lotions any time. Okay?"

"For just a minute. I don't want my skin to dry out. Bed sores can happen very quickly."

I stretched out in my sleeping space and slowly counted backward from one hundred, commanding my body to loosen the knots.

"Don't go to sleep, Mom. Let's get through with the lotions."

When I tried to discourage such a meticulous and lengthy routine, he would say, "I've got to do the best I can. Everybody has to do their part. This is my part. It's the only thing I can do."

He was still being given morphine round the clock and I began to doubt its effectiveness. I wondered if he knew what he was doing or saying. Once he scrubbed his face so hard, he made it irritated. A doctor who came by and saw the red splotches immediately called for a nurse to take his temperature. Each time I tried to restrain him from the rigorous scrubbing, he said over and over, "This is my part. I've got to do the best I can."

Even in his pain and euphoric world of morphine, he dictated exactly where each item was to be placed at his bedside, in the order he might need to reach it. He insisted that the wastebasket be placed exactly where all he had to do was reach his hand over the side of the bed and drop something.

About every thirty minutes, he called out, "Mom, give me some water. And please fix it right this time."

"Here you are. How does this look?"

With bleary eyes, he slowly inspected the cup and said, "It needs more ice. Don't you have any more ice? You know I like it filled to the top with water."

"I don't want you to spill it."

"I'm not going to spill it! Put more water in it. Will you ever learn how to bend the straw? It has to be bent exactly right or it'll drip. Fix it again...get another straw...."

When I could be objective, I found it interesting that he would make such paramount issues of insignificant things. It appeared he was grasping for anything to hold on to, to keep his sanity in his ordeal of torture. I wondered how an analyst might have identified the force behind his insistence on perfection in these minute details.

While facing a seemingly insurmountable problem and experiencing excruciating pain, he focused on little things he could have control over. He couldn't control the big problem so he majored on the minor ones. I supposed it was normal.

∾

Dr. Cook, who had assisted Dr. Malawer, visited twice each day and the nurses seemed to be in awe of him as he barked out orders and requested things they didn't have on the floor. It didn't take long to recognize that this surgeon wasn't accustomed to working with oncology nurses. The floor wasn't equipped with things surgeons needed.

Earlier in the week when Dr. Cook was examining Ross's leg, I asked about the black areas on his foot. They hadn't changed.

He said, "That's called 'necrosis'."

The cast had been put on improperly and was too tight on his foot. The black "stuff" was actually dead, "necrotic" skin and tissue.

The agonizing pain Ross experienced encircled his entire leg and foot. He couldn't know that the pain in his foot wasn't caused by the surgery on his leg. Morphine hadn't relieved his pain, but had clouded his senses. From Thursday night until late Sunday afternoon, a gripping vise had been clamped on his foot, becoming tighter and tighter as the area swelled under the cast. Now, the skin and tissue were dead.

I recalled seeing Dr. Malawer on the telephone after he removed the cast. He had appeared unhappy about something, and now I knew why. How I wished I had demanded of someone to look at Ross's leg when he cried out so pitifully. I thought all the pain was caused by the removal of bone in his leg. I went into the bathroom, closed the door, leaned my forehead on the wall and cried. Dealing with cancer was enough. He shouldn't have to deal with human failure.

On Wednesday, it was decided that he needed a blood transfusion. He had been given blood during surgery and now, almost a week after surgery, his blood counts indicated he needed more. He had no bleeding since surgery but he looked jaundiced. His facial hair had not completely fallen out and he had a gray shadow from not shaving. Dark circles ringed his eyes.

I had told Ross that he was going to have a visitor. A man from Alabama, Jo Bonner, former staff member of Congressman Callahan's office, was in town and had invited me to lunch.

When Jo arrived, he nervously stood by the bed and tried to chat with Ross. Soon I said, "Let's go, you promised me lunch."

"We don't have to do that if you think you shouldn't leave," he said softly, as he glanced at Ross.

"No deal, Josiah, let's go," I insisted.

With Jo dressed in a well-cut suit, buttoned-down shirt with a striped tie, and me in sneakers, blue jeans, and an old silk blouse, we walked out to the elevator.

"I don't think you should get far away from the hospital, Elaine. Let's stay here and go to the cafeteria."

"No way. I've got to get out of here and I need to check on a hotel room. I have to get some sleep." Tears rose to my eyes.

"Okay, where do you want to go?"

"Let's go to the Marriott. I can check on a room and they have a nice family-style restaurant,—that is, if you're not too embarrassed about the way I look."

After lunch, I checked at the Marriott desk for a room but there was nothing available. Jo drove me back to the hospital where we said goodbye in front of the building.

When I entered the lobby, I walked straight to a telephone and called around for a place to stay. I found a room at a little inn in Bethesda where I had stayed before. It wasn't very good, but it mattered little, I thought, as long as there was a bed. I reserved the room for three nights and guaranteed it.

The blood transfusion was finished when I walked back in the room and Ross had perked up a bit.

"Where did you go?" he asked.

"Allie's Pantry at the Marriott."

"What did you have to eat?"

"Chicken salad with cantaloupe," I said, thankful he didn't care for either.

"I wish I could go somewhere and have a nice lunch. I get hungry, too, and the food around here is the pits."

I should have brought him something.

When I called home to give Bill the hotel phone number, Scott came on the line and reminded me that he was going to move to Huntsville, Alabama, during the next few days. He had dropped out of school until he could decide exactly what he wanted to study.

I would miss him. He and I had become very close during the past five years while he groped his way through some of the anxieties that plagued him. He was still in the process of overcoming some hurdles, and I knew this move to Huntsville would take courage.

"Could you maybe postpone this until I get home and we can talk more about it?" I asked.

"No, Mom, there's nothing to discuss. The time's right and I need to go ahead."

"I'm sorry I'm not there to help send you off. Promise to keep in close touch."

"I will, Mom. I'll call you when I get settled."

"I'm really going to miss you, Scott. I love you."

"Love you, too, Mom. Don't worry about me."

That evening, I nervously told Ross that I had taken a room in a motel on Wisconsin Avenue but I would stay with him as late as he wanted and be back early in the morning.

He looked unhappy.

"You'll be okay, honey. Don't worry, the nurses take good care of you. They always come quickly when you call."

"Not always, they don't."

"I really need to get some sleep. I've not had any rest," I said.

"I haven't either, you know."

"Don't the sleeping pills work, at least for a little while?"

"No, they don't. Nothing works."

"I'm leaving the motel phone number at the nurses' station, so if you need me they can call me. I can be back in ten minutes."

At 9:00 p.m., I placed a few things in an overnight bag and walked out of the room. I was hungry, so I went to the hospital cafeteria for a piece of egg custard pie and a carton of milk to take to the motel. My appetite was gone when I went into my room, but I noticed a small dorm-type refrigerator and thought I would save my food until later. Opening the refrigerator door, I confronted someone else's old food, along with a huge dead bug. Food forgotten, I fell into the bed.

Early the next morning, I hastily showered, dressed, and took all my things with me back to the hospital. Although I had reserved the room for three nights, I didn't know if I would make it back.

Ross was awake when I walked into the room.

"Did you sleep well?" he asked.

"Sure did. What about you?"

"No, I didn't sleep at all. I wish I could go to a hotel."

This day was like all the others—constant pain and continuing morphine. The Port-A-Cath served its intended purpose. All medications were put through the IV, which had been there since surgery. Ross's vital signs were closely monitored. The fever that he'd had since Monday persisted.

Dr. Cook visited twice that day, as he normally did, and he told Ross about the planned graft for the next day. Skin would be taken from his left thigh to be placed over the exposed area of the surgery site. The wound had been kept padded with wet dressings to prepare it to receive the grafts.

All day, Ross issued orders, and I failed to execute them as he wished. The pillows weren't placed properly, the bed wasn't elevated or lowered to his liking, the sheets became crumpled because I didn't tuck them in tight enough, or there was something he needed and couldn't reach. The bath and lotion routine continued. Again, I left him and returned to the motel. With key in hand, I went directly to the room with my overnight bag. Wearily, I walked in and placed my bag on the bed.

It took a few minutes to register on my brain that the shower was running and the bathroom door was closed. In the closet by the door I had just entered was a man's jacket, shoes and a suitcase. Grabbing my things, I sailed out of the room. When I reached the front desk in the lobby, I found a lady who hardly spoke English.

"But you check out," she said.

"No, I did not check out!" I said. "Why did you put that man in my room? I still have my key. See?"

"But you left. You take all your things. I check it myself."

"I did not check out. Give me another room and let's stop arguing about it."

"We have no nother room, I think," she said.

"Where is the manager? I want to speak to the desk manager."

"They all gone. I'm only one here."

"Look at the reservation. See, it says for three nights. I suggest you find the manager and telephone him."

I must have intimidated her, for she remembered there was a suite of rooms which was three times more expensive. She said I could have it for the night, one night only.

The "suite,"—an elongated room with a kitchen at one end— was a bit cleaner than other rooms I had stayed in.

Again, I fell asleep immediately. Before I caught the shuttle to the hospital early the next morning, I stopped by the desk and told them what had happened the night before. They assured me I would have a room for that night, but not the suite I had been in. They had done me a big favor by letting me stay in the suite at the same price as the regular room.

The gurney was in the hall outside Ross's room when I arrived. Ross was staring at the door. "How was your night?" he asked. "Is the motel nice?"

"It's okay. I wouldn't pick it for a vacation spot, but it serves the purpose."

"What took you so long to get here? I'm about to go to surgery."

"Heavy traffic and a late shuttle. It's only seven-thirty. I'm not really late."

"I've been expecting you for an hour."

"Do you need me to do something for you?"

"Not anymore, I don't. I had to ask someone else to help me. I guess you had a nice breakfast."

"No, Ross, I didn't even have coffee. I'll get it later."

Soon four orderlies lifted the blanket under him and slowly placed him on the gurney. I walked to the elevator with them, and again the car was waiting.

At the surgery door, I squeezed his hand and kissed him on the forehead. As I walked away, I wished someone other than Dr. Cook was doing the skin grafts, possibly a plastic surgeon. Dr. Cook had been around for a long time and was an excellent man in his field, but he and I didn't communicate very well.

Not long after surgery, he volunteered the discouraging news that the pathology report on the bone removed from Ross's leg indicated that the three rounds of chemotherapy hadn't been as effective as they had hoped. I saw no reason to give Ross this disheartening report, considering that he faced many more dismal months of treatment.

Since Dr. Cook wasn't an oncologist, I wondered why he felt it was his place to be the one to convey this message. Perhaps it was appropriate for him to give us the report; however, often it seemed that he took opportunities to boost his own specialty at the expense of the oncologists.

I thought he was pompous and snobbish. He seemed to talk down to Ross and me. Since I had asked about the necrotic places on Ross's foot, he had acted very defensive. Anything we questioned was answered with abrupt, flippant responses. Also, when he left the room, I felt he had placed the blame on Ross or me for whatever complaint Ross had. I didn't like him.

He was one of the first surgeons who walked through the examining room in September, 1982, when we first arrived at NIH. Even then, he showed no patience with me or Ross. He presented himself as being loftier than us mortals, often reminding me that he was a *surgeon*. Looking back, I didn't like his attitude then.

It must be my fault. He must be good. He'd been there a long time. I hadn't heard any other patients complain about him but I didn't know if other patients on the hall had ever had any experience with him. It really made no difference what I thought of him as long as he did a good job taking care of Ross.

Ross wasn't in surgery very long, and was soon back in his room. The left thigh, where the five-inch strips of skin had been taken, had bright red pieces of gauze over the donor sites. The gauze strips seemed to be stuck since there was no tape holding them. This surgery immobilized him even more.

It also necessitated more equipment in the already packed space on Ross's side of the room. A sunlamp was brought in to be used on the donor site several times a day. The surgical site where the grafts were placed had been bandaged, not to be opened for one week.

The left thigh burned intensely, but the morphine had never stopped, so Ross's complaints were no more than usual. The skin graft site and the new area of trauma on the left thigh complicated the bath and lotion routine because it had to be left untouched. Ross had to remain absolutely flat on his back.

Late that evening, I left him again and returned to the motel, not knowing what to expect. In fact, I did have a room—but the door wouldn't close completely tight. I hooked a chain and propped a chair under the door knob. I fell into bed.

Sometime after midnight, I woke to screaming and yelling in the room next door. In near panic, I sat up and listened to a big fight with crashing noises that sounded like furniture being tossed around and something, or someone, bouncing against my wall. I turned the light on and reached for the phone to call the desk. There was no dial tone. Looking more carefully, I saw that the phone was broken and, in fact, wasn't even hooked up.

The fight spilled out of the room and into the parking lot outside my door. On tiptoe, I looked out the peephole as someone screeched by, followed by a thud against a car fender. Voices got louder and I prayed someone would wake up—someone who had a telephone that worked.

I was trapped. There was nothing I could do. I turned the light off, covered my head with a pillow, and prayed that no one would come crashing through the wall. After a few minutes, I heard sirens. With a grateful heart, I drifted back to sleep.

When I awoke the next morning, I wondered how I would respond to Ross's questions about my night in the motel. I didn't want to admit that I would have gotten more rest if I had stayed at the hospital.

When I checked out, I promised myself I would never return. But I did.

29

October, 1988

At 3:00 a.m., I awoke in my bunk bed, the drape pulled around me. I heard a nurse whispering softly to Ross, "Try to stop thinking about the future, your hopes and plans. Make the best of the situation now, in the present moment. We're here. We love you. Don't shut us out." I couldn't hear Ross's whispered response.

His primary nurse and one of the social workers went into the District to hear Dr. Siegel speak, and they brought Ross a copy of Dr. Siegel's meditation tape. He was pleased to hear *Canon in D*—the background music for Dr. Siegel's voice. Often he fell asleep with the earphones on.

Because Ross and I were reading Dr. Siegel's book, some people thought we were groping for an illusive lifeline. But until it is known exactly how our immune systems work and why the control for cell division sometimes fails to function, anything was worth investigating if it didn't interfere with established medical practices. It couldn't hurt, and it might help.

I had heard some doctors and ministers say that certain books or religious beliefs and practices gave false hope. Nevertheless, I thought it was better than no hope. Since real hope had become clouded, the choices left were no hope or false hope. Hope was essential to recovery. And until it could be proven false, who could say that it was? Who could deny that hope, even if based on a seemingly false premise, could trigger some mysterious bodily mechanism which would boost the immune system and correct the cell division? Could some component of the immune system have intelligence? Could it differentiate between real and false hope? How would it respond to despair? Would it react at all to either one?

Late one afternoon when Ross was particularly depressed and in pain, I searched for an expression of hope and encouragement, trying to come up with new words, new thoughts. He was exhausted but couldn't get comfortable enough to go to sleep.

I decided to try my newly-found and little-practiced "grateful heart" attitude on him. It was all I had left.

"You have a new pillow under your head. Does it feel good?"

"Yes, it's a lot better than that 'ratty' one."

"Can you possibly say, 'Thank you, God'?"

He lay still, but moved his eyes to look at me, questioning.

"Let's try something. Starting with where you are right now, let's think of all the things you have to be grateful for. Don't think about anything bad—just think good things." My words sounded more appropriate for a small child and I expected a retort from him. But he listened.

"We can be thankful that, under these circumstances, you are here, in this place. Thank God you've not been shot, lying wounded, alone, in a muddy ditch in a war zone in a foreign country. Or in a back alley of a slum in a strange city."

He looked out the window toward a patch of blue sky.

"You can be thankful for the ice in the cup, for the drinks in the fridge down the hall. Look at all the neat little inventions and designs of things you need. Someone developed everything from the straw in the glass to that headset you listen to. Think of all the books you have—the hours and hours that went into writing and publishing them."

He stretched out a bit and twisted to a more comfortable position.

"Think of this place, the nurses—how great they are and how much they love you. The talent of the doctors, all the equipment —just think about how much brainpower went into creating this place."

He snuggled down in his pillow, yawned, and pulled a sheet up under his chin.

"Somewhere in the Bible there's a place called Bethesda. It was a pool where people went when they needed healing. Even for that, we can have a grateful heart. You're in a place of healing."

When I looked down at him, his eyes were closed and he was breathing evenly. He had drifted off somewhere between the roses blooming in front of the building and "the place of healing waters."

That's the first step, I thought. Later, we'll talk about the next step—keeping a grateful heart even at times when there is nothing we can see to be thankful for. We'll try to be thankful *in spite of.*

While wondering how to approach Ross with the second step, and when reflecting on his past, I realized that, on some level, he had been doing this all along, unaware of any other way.

The next morning, his cousin, Allan Riorda, called from Baltimore and asked if he could come down to visit. Thank God, I thought. I urged him to be on his way. In the recreation room, I found a big TV on rollers and pushed it into Ross's room. Allan was still a big New Orleans Saints' football fan.

Allan, sandy-haired and handsome, was three years older than Ross. Wearing jeans and a Saints' sweatshirt, he leaned forward toward the TV and immediately entered the spirit of the game, yelling and swinging his arms, second-guessing the coaches, and cheering the Saints on. His antics and his running commentary made Ross laugh—a first in a long time.

"Why don't you take a break, Aunt Elaine?" Allan asked. "I'll look after him."

"Gladly," I said. I picked up my purse and left, knowing the game would last at least two or three hours. When I reached the downstairs lobby, I headed for the front door. I wanted to get outside. But, as I walked through the gallery, I looked in the distance toward the entrance and realized my legs could move no more. I could go no farther.

The large, stuffed lounge chairs along the walkway through the gallery pulled at me like a magnet. I sat, and in a few seconds, I leaned my head over the arm of the chair.

Three hours later, I woke with a searing pain in my rib cage. People walked by, talking, inches from my chair. Music came from somewhere. I didn't know where I was. Slowly, I looked around, rubbed my eyes and remembered. I returned to the 13th floor in time to say goodbye to Allan.

Mary took me out to dinner one night and, while in the restaurant, my chest and ribs hurt so badly I had to leave the table. She said, "Mom, something has to change. You need a long break—not just a night or two in a hotel. You need to go home."

My exhaustion seemed evident to everyone—even a stranger on an elevator. I had seen the elevator operator many times, often when Ross was going to surgery. Another passenger was already on the elevator when I stepped on, a foreign-looking woman dressed in a silk sari. She eyed me carefully.

"How's your boy?" the operator asked.

"He's okay. He's going to be all right."

"He sure has been through a lot."

"Yes, he has."

"Must be mighty rough on you."

"Yes, sometimes it is," I said.

The other passenger had remained silent during this exchange as we continued down. Suddenly, she smiled brightly and said, "*Vy...don...you...go...hom?*"

Without thinking, I said to her, "It's too far away."

But even after realizing how far she'd had to travel, I couldn't muster up any gratitude for being only a thousand miles away from home.

Five days after the skin graft, the bandages were removed and the site examined. It wasn't a 100-percent "take" but Dr. Cook seemed pleased.

As I watched the bandages being changed on Ross's leg, I had noticed a tiny spot that was a strange color. Neither white, gray, pink, nor yellow, it seemed to be a combination of those hues. It was barely below the surface of the skin, about one-quarter inch long. The spot was in one of the incision lines where other odd-looking, pink and brown scabs were, and it looked curious among all the other things. I asked Dr. Cook if it could possibly be a small infected area.

He smirked at my ignorance and said, "We'd know if there was an infection. It's probably just a scab that hasn't completely formed."

Later, when he and Dr. Malawer came in together to look at the site, nothing was said about the strange-looking spot. Dr. Malawer asked Ross to try to wiggle his toes. After a few seconds of concentration, he moved his big toe, looked up at me, and smiled like a little boy.

Two weeks after surgery, three nurses placed their arms and hands in position and lifted him to a chair beside his bed, but it was too painful to sit. However, each day they continued to insist he try again, extending his time of tolerance. After searching the entire hospital, they found a special wheelchair that would accommodate his leg, and I pushed him along the hall, into the elevator, and out of the building.

Outside by the cafeteria, a half-block long sidewalk slants down toward the street. When I pushed the chair through the door of the cafeteria, Ross grabbed the wheel with his right hand and pushed furiously until he gained momentum and rolled all the way down the hill to the street.

He had been depressed and cross with everyone that day. It wasn't easy to be around him. I started walking down the incline to catch up with him, but then changed my mind. He would have to figure out how to get back up the hill with only one hand to roll the wheelchair. I sat down by a picnic table.

He sat looking along the street for a long time, then maneuvered the chair in position to return. He pushed forward, then rolled back. Again he pushed, sticking his leg out to try to stop the backward motion. He heaved forward, running the wheels off the walk and onto the grass.

Restraining my impulse to go to him, I leaned over, tied my

shoes and picked up some acorns, carefully examining them. Out of the corner of my eye, I could see that he had progressed only about five feet up the incline.

He wiped his eyes and nose with his shirt sleeve. People walked hurriedly past him and he turned his head away. Leaning forward, he lunged with determination, quickly moving his hand back and grabbing the wheel to keep the hard-won advance. Even though it was a chilly day, I knew he was sweating.

Turning my back, I opened my purse and retrieved a note pad with my list of reminders. I checked off a few and added more. When I turned to look at him, I saw that he was halfway up the hill. The chair was turned sideways and his back was toward me. I rose and slowly strolled in his direction.

"Want some help?" I asked.

"I'm resting," he said.

"I can push if you're tired."

"No."

Biting his lip, he leaned forward, pushing hard over the last mound before the walk leveled. He was drenched with sweat and his face was drained of color. "Open the door, please. I want to go in."

The crush of lunch customers carrying food trays brought him to a complete standstill. "Let me push the chair through this crowd," I said.

"Walk in front of me. I'll do it."

We maneuvered through the cafeteria and along the hall towards the elevator. When it arrived, I stepped aside so he could enter.

"Get on, Mom. Move to the back so I can turn around."

He was silent until we reached the 13th floor. As I held the heavy hall door opened and he pushed through, I said, "You did good, Ross."

"I've got to do the best I can."

❧

Three weeks after surgery, he was allowed to stand by the bed for a few minutes. The crutches were brought out of the closet and the IV was unhooked for the first time.

On Monday, another angel appeared. Marti Weiss from Potomac, Maryland, had graduated from Spring Hill College a year before Ross. Marti had personal, first-hand experience with cancer and was doing well after her surgery a few years before at another hospital. A tall, pretty, vibrant, strong and healthy girl with luxurious long, dark hair, Marti visited Ross in the evenings after she got off from work. She helped him learn how to use the crutches without bending his knee while she supported him with her arm around his waist. Unrelenting in her demands, she tolerated no depressing talk. She was loving, affectionate, and patient with him. She also knew when to leave him alone.

Marti now lived in an apartment near Rockville, and her roommate, Joy, was an oncology nurse at Sibley Hospital. Since they passed the NIH on their way home from work, they ran errands for Ross and brought him special suppers.

Another unanticipated gift came in the form of a volunteer on the 13th floor. She had a full time job, yet devoted her Monday evenings to volunteering at the nurses' station. A middle-aged, professional woman, her career with the Central Intelligence Agency and related activities at the State Department seemed especially designed for Ross. When she learned of Ross's interest in foreign affairs, she visited him and, thereafter, her time on the hall was spent by his bed. He looked forward to Monday evenings. In addition to providing an intellectual stimulus for him, she kept his dream alive that he would someday work in the field of foreign relations.

A well-dressed, gracious library volunteer went beyond the call of her duty. She pushed a cart along the halls with a variety of reading materials, going into each patient's room to ask if he or she would like something to read. Each time she asked Ross, he always said, "No, thank you."

One day, when she asked if there was anything specific he

would like, Ross said, "I'm so dopey, I can't concentrate. I doubt I could read anything more than a comic book."

"That's fine," she said. "I'll get you some comic books. What kind do you like?"

Ross thought for a moment and said, "I like *Calvin and Hobbes*. I used to like *Doonesbury*. I don't think the library has any of those."

She shopped for Ross's comic books and brought them to him.

These angels of mercy eased Ross through the unending days of pain and hospital routines. They were a welcome relief from the constant parade of doctors, nurses, technicians and other staff who were in the room.

Each time Dr. Cook came in, he looked at Ross's damaged foot and examined his leg while removing bits of dead skin from the edges. He obviously wasn't afraid of AIDS, since he never wore gloves and used his fingers to pick out the pieces of dead skin. Again, I asked about the peculiar-looking spot in the incision line. He told me to ignore it. It was nothing.

Days went by with the same routine until the morning when a construction worker walked into Ross's and Tommy's room and announced that both of them would soon have to be moved out in order for some work to be done on the ceiling. They would each be placed with another patient. Ross hoped to be put with little Mark Daullary, but learned that Mark already had a room-mate, so we moved to the end of the hall.

But Mark often came to visit Ross on days when he felt like getting out of bed. Wearing his baseball cap slightly askew, push-ing his IV pole, he quietly eased into Ross's room, stood near the bed and watched as the bandages and dressings were changed. His thin, frail body with its pale skin revealed the ravages of his disease and treatment. As he silently observed all the activity around Ross's bed, his already large eyes seemed even bigger because of the dark shadows around them. As soon as the nurses left the room, he would talk to Ross, but he had little to say to anyone else. Ross tried to encourage Mark to eat, and he talked to him about how great it was going to be when he got out of the hospital—all the fun things he could do at home.

Although Ross tried to hide his own feelings when around

Mark, one day his distress reached a new high. Not long after Mark had left the room, Dr. Cook walked in and found Ross crying. "I've got to get out of here! I can't stand much more of this," he said.

Dr. Cook said, "Stop feeling sorry for yourself. You've not been here as long as a lot of patients have. Buck up! Get tough with yourself. You're not ready to go home."

Here he goes again, I thought, trying to make Ross feel guilty. "Is it out of the question for him to get a pass for the weekend so I can take him to a hotel?" I asked.

The doctor continued to use his fingernails as he picked at the edge of the grafts and around the necrotic area. "I doubt you can manage this by yourself, but if you insist, go ahead! I'll discharge him," he said. He gave me a cold stare and stalked out the door.

After I shot visual arrows into his back, I picked up the phone and called all the motels and little inns in the area. Finally, I found a room available—at the inn where I had sworn never to return. I took it, glad that I had not told Ross about my escapades.

Mary was out of town and I wondered how I could manage this dubious gift of freedom alone. We had over a month's collection of things to be thrown into suitcases and bags. I cleared Ross's bulletin board of all his greeting cards, gathered up all his clothes and books, and started packing.

Marti called. I told her our good news and that I might need her Saturday morning to help us move to a different hotel. The Marriott had space for Saturday and Sunday nights.

Ross didn't care what the motel was like. He was finally out. I carried sterile sheets, surgical instruments, dressings and gauzes, sterile water, urinals, and medicines. I managed the dressings and medications by myself that night. A deli was nearby and Ross kept me running back and forth to the little shop to find specific things he thought he might like to eat.

Saturday morning, Marti arrived in her small car. She was going to take Ross for a drive and then to the Marriott while I followed in a taxi with all our things.

When we got Ross out to Marti's car, we discovered that he wouldn't fit in the front seat because he couldn't bend his knee. Her car was a two-door, so she crawled into the back and lifted him into the seat, pushing the front seat forward and folding it down. They drove off with Ross in the back seat with his leg propped on the folded front seat. He made a funny face at me, smiled, and waved as they turned the corner and entered the traffic on Wisconsin Avenue.

Soon after I reached our room at the Marriott, the two of them came slowly along the hall—Marti with her arm around Ross as she supported him on crutches. When they entered the room, they both collapsed on the bed.

The manager of the pool brought two lounge chairs and placed them outside our room on the little terrace. I walked to a deli on Pooks Hill Road and bought food for a picnic lunch. Marti and Ross sat side by side in the sunlight, eating their sandwiches while listening to his favorite tapes.

"Glad to be here, huh?" Marti teased, as she leaned over to kiss him on his cheek.

"I've never been so glad in my whole life...Oh, man...."

Marti said something to him in a low voice, and they both broke up in laughter—real laughter from Ross.

I reentered the room and closed the sliding glass door. I could faintly hear their music as they rocked side-to-side in time with the beat. They sang along with the lyrics.

Marti helped me change the dressings twice that day, using sterile procedures. She was adept at assisting and knew the importance of using sterile water and freshly opened tweezers for each change.

Late that afternoon after she left, Ross seemed depressed. "Someone else has to come up here, Mom. You've got to go home. Haven't you been here almost three weeks?" Tears formed in his eyes.

He had lost track of time. I had been there five weeks.

"Can't Dad come up? What about Aunt Jean?" he asked.

"Jean has a job and two teenage boys in school, Ross. She can't come. Let's don't ask her."

"Call Dad. See if he'll come," he said. "You can't take this anymore. You're going to get sick and then what? Go home, take a break. I need a break from you, Mom," he said, with quivering lips.

"We both need a break from each other. I know that. But I don't know what we can do about it."

His shoulders began to shake and he buried his face in his hand. "You can come back when I have the thoracotomy," he said.

We needed a road map so we could clearly see and know how to plan. The chemotherapy was originally scheduled to begin about this time, but with the necrotic foot, scheduled skin grafts, and the planned thoracotomy, nothing had been said about chemo. Physical therapy, vitally important after his leg surgery, hadn't even been mentioned. He didn't have a schedule anymore.

I remembered hearing Dr. Malawer and Dr. Cook discussing Ross's surgery site and how good it looked. "Don't say that too loud," one of them said. "The oncologists might hear you and decide it's time to start treatment." It was then that I knew there was a difference of opinion between the two branches, and Ross was a topic of many discussions in conference. It appeared that the oncologists thought the treatment should not be delayed and surgical procedures should be planned around their schedule. The surgeons thought the treatment should be worked around their planned procedures and therapy.

On Sunday morning, Ross sat in bed staring at the TV. I placed his room-service breakfast on a tray beside him. He turned to me and asked, "Have you figured out what you'll do?"

"About what?"

"I told you. I want you to go home."

"No, I haven't figured that out. I don't know what to do. You can't take care of yourself yet, and I don't think I should walk off and leave you."

"I don't care how you do it, but I want you to leave."

"You're beginning to upset me, Ross. You're hurting my feelings."

"That's just the point. It's enough to have to deal with my own feelings. I can't worry about yours. That's your problem, not mine. I appreciate all the stuff you've done for me, but it's my life and I can tell you I want you to go home."

"What's the matter? What have I done to make you so angry?"

"I'm not angry with you. I'm just ready for you to leave."

"And who's going to take care of you?" I asked, as I turned and looked out the window.

"You figure it out. Find somebody and then you go home."

We had little to say to each other for the rest of the day. Late Sunday afternoon, he said he didn't feel well and we checked his temperature. It was slightly elevated. When changing the dressing that night, I saw a slight change in a spot on the edge of the necrotic area. It looked a little inflamed.

I dialed our home number, and, when Bill answered, I handed the phone to Ross. Ross tearfully asked him to please come up. Bill told him he would have to go to the office the next day and take care of some things, but would come up Tuesday. I was to leave Wednesday.

This news eased the tension between us. Both of us were too exhausted to even argue about anything anymore. He continued to take his pain medication but also said he didn't feel well. Another check of his temperature revealed a slightly higher elevation, but still below 100 degrees.

The next morning, first thing, he asked me to look at his foot. Sure enough, there it was—a spot of infection. His temperature hovered near 100. I called the clinic and told them we were on our way.

While Ross was in the examination room, Dr. Cook appeared in the waiting room and announced to me and everyone else who was there, "I tried to tell you that you couldn't take care of him properly in a hotel room."

I bit my tongue. But I wanted to scream at him and say, "Keep your fingernails away from his leg and foot, you jerk!" I remembered the horrible staph infection when the catheter lines were changed during the summer. I could hardly be blamed for that, since no one touched the site except the professionals.

I was incredulous when I fully realized that he had walked all the way from the examination room to the waiting room to make his speech.

Ross was returned to the 13th floor and the IV antibiotics restarted. That night I went back to the hotel and wept. I wondered if Dr. Cook was correct in his assessment of my nursing ability. He had been completely successful in shaking what little confidence

I had and in making me feel worthless. Slowly, I began to pack for my trip home.

Bill arrived on Tuesday, and I tried to brief him on the requirements for his role as primary caregiver. But there was too much to tell, so he would have to learn as he went along day by day.

On my way to the hospital Wednesday morning, I prepared myself to say good-bye. When I went into Ross's room, I began to feel teary and had to leave. I went to the watts line in the hall and phoned my friend, Sally Green, to tell her it wasn't necessary for her to meet me at the airport in Mobile as she had offered, because Bill had left my car there for me. She said she'd like to meet me anyway.

Neither Ross nor I could say good-bye. A couple of nurses had tears in their eyes as they watched our efforts. Then, someone said something humorous and all of us started laughing, somewhat hysterically, wiping our tears away. I walked away.

During the drive through the countryside from Maryland to the airport, I felt as if I had been released from prison. The sunlight seemed brighter; the trees were reds, yellows, and golds.

As the plane lifted off the runway, my eyes filled with tears. We passed over the Lincoln Memorial, and I looked out the window at the Capitol and other familiar monuments as they came into view. I continued to watch for landmarks, and saw the National Cathedral near Chevy Chase. In the distance, I could see the spires of the Mormon Church. Although the sun was shining, there were threatening, dark clouds gathering.

I looked down, and there it was—the sprawling red brick building of the Clinic Center on the campus of NIH.

With my forehead pressed against the glass in the window, I gazed at the hospital. Before it left my field of vision, I lifted my head and looked high in the sky above the hospital. And there, I saw a rainbow. That's mine, I thought. That rainbow is for me.

∾

"Welcome home," Sally said, hugging me.

"I'm beyond conversation—forgive me," I said.

"It's okay. Give me your car keys."

Blonde, petite Sally acted like a stevedore. She loaded my luggage in the trunk, then followed me home, again moving all my bags into the house. When we arrived at my side door, there was a big basket of fresh flowers sitting at the entrance.

"Well, well. Look what you have here," Sally said.

"It may be a mistake. Few people knew I was coming home. I don't think anyone would send flowers."

I put the pretty basket on the table and opened the attached envelope. It said, "Welcome home, Mom. I love you. Ross."

In a few minutes, the phone rang. "Mom? Welcome home."

"Ross! You okay?"

"I'm okay. What about you? Did you have a good flight?"

"Everything went fine. Sally met me and followed me home."

"Have you seen Mitty, Maggie, Mikey, and Max?"

"There were a few cats around but I don't know which ones. I just got here, just a few minutes ago."

"Anything else going on?"

"Let me think...Oh yes, someone sent me some flowers."

"Really?"

"They're beautiful, Ross. How did you manage that?"

"Don't worry about it."

"I'm going to miss you, buddy."

"I miss you already, Mom. But I'm glad you're home. Get some rest."

"I will. I love you, Ross."

"Love you, too, Mom. Bye."

30

Dressings on Ross's foot were changed every four hours each day, and the areas of trauma began to slowly shed the necrotic skin. On top of his foot on the curve of the instep, and on the back of his heel, there were spots which resisted healing. There was a tiny hole on the instep, and when Ross moved his toe, a wiggling tendon could be seen down in the opening. This was a continuous avenue for infection, just inches from the implant in his leg.

Skin grafts over this spot weren't successful and suturing it wasn't possible. As the surgeons had explained to me while I was still there, the skin and tissue in that area were like cheese and wouldn't hold a suture. All efforts to close the hole were unsuccessful.

On Thursday, Bill called at my office to tell me that the surgeons were planning to cut the tendon which controlled the movement of the big toe. It wouldn't affect his walking ability, but the toe would most likely droop and he wouldn't be able to move it again—a relatively insignificant addition to his mounting load of problems.

Bill had spent the last week and a half of October with Ross, then returned to Mobile, leaving Ross alone for the weekend with Mary checking up on him. I made a plane reservation to go up the following Wednesday for the thoracotomy on Thursday. Late Tuesday afternoon, Ross telephoned me.

"Mom? I've got some news—the thoracotomy has been canceled," he said.

I didn't detect any excitement in his voice. "Canceled? Why? What happened?"

"Dr. Pass, the surgeon who does thoracotomies, looked at the X-rays and said he didn't think it was a nodule and we shouldn't do the surgery."

"That's wonderful! Thank God! Isn't that great?"

"I guess so. I just hope he's right."

"Isn't he the one who does most all the thoracotomies up there? Shouldn't he know better than anyone if it's a nodule?"

"I guess so. I don't know anything anymore," Ross sighed, his voice sounding weak and distant.

"It's been hanging over your head for six weeks. Can you relax a little?"

"I don't know, Mom. I don't know what to think."

"If Dr. Pass thinks it's not a nodule, what does he think it is?"

"Nobody knows. They said it may be caused by a virus or an infection I've had."

"The neckline catheter! Remember that awful experience with the staph infection? That has to be it."

"Whatever. I'm just glad I don't have to have my chest cut open and my ribs pulled apart," he whispered.

I canceled my reservations.

He remained in the hospital with continued dressing changes on his foot and little else going on. The hole in his foot didn't close, even after clipping the tendon.

The following Tuesday, November 8th, was election day in Mobile. Mr. Callahan won the race comfortably and Bill and I attended his celebration party that evening. But my thoughts weren't on the election returns that night.

The chemotherapy treatments were now about four weeks overdue. In order for Ross to be a part of the study, he had to follow the protocol. Otherwise his treatment results couldn't be considered in the final analysis.

While Bill and I were at the election party in Mobile, an oncologist Ross didn't know well had floor duty. He came by to visit Ross, and somewhere in the conversation the word "amputation" was mentioned. Ross surmised they were discussing the possibility of amputating his leg in order to get back on chemotherapy.

Early the next morning, he asked for the psychiatric nurse to come to see him. After Jacques left, Ross called me. He was very upset, but firm in his voice when he told me he thought amputation was being considered. He told me the name of the doctor who had dropped this bomb on him.

"Who's he? I've never heard of him. Is he new? You're not his patient. I'm calling Stacey Berg right now."

"Let me know what she says."

"I'm coming up there, Ross. They're not going to treat you this way. How dare they even think this!"

"Call Dr. Berg and see what she says."

I did. She said she would have to find out who had floor duty the night before. Although she was non-committal, I knew that somewhere, sometime, somebody had brought up the subject of amputation. The new doctor possibly thought Ross had already been told. I told Dr. Berg I would be up there the next day and wanted to meet with whoever was making decisions.

When I walked along the hall of the 13th floor of NIH at noon the next day, Dr. Berg and the night doctor were waiting for me. They walked toward me with apologies.

"I didn't mean to upset Ross," the young doctor said. "We were just chatting about his long delay in getting treatment and a lot of different possibilities. I'm sorry if I said the wrong thing."

"Yes, you said the wrong thing," I said, as I continued toward Ross's room.

It had been three weeks since I left, and 12 days since Bill returned home. When I walked in and looked at Ross, he seemed hardly to have moved. When he hugged me tightly as I leaned over the bed, I saw a little moisture form in his eyes, but it quickly went away.

"What's going on? Anything new?" I asked.

"No. My foot still has a hole in it. Either I'm getting used to the pain or I'm getting better, because my leg doesn't hurt as bad as it did. I can read a little now and keep up with what's going on in the world."

"What are you reading?"

"The *Post* mainly. *The New York Times* when I can get it. Sometimes *U.S. News*. Mark's dad brings me the *Post* every day. The recreation staff bring me movies for the VCR from wherever they can find them. I've seen about a hundred movies, I think."

He switched the conversation to his favorite subject—the political changes and climate in various parts of the world. He asked me questions I couldn't answer, and was impatient with my lack of awareness of up-to-the-minute world events.

"What's going on at home? Any important mail for me? Any of my friends call?"

"I've brought your mail and a list of people who have called asking about you. Not much else is going on. Mr. Callahan won the election."

"I knew that—saw it on NBC. How's the weather down there? How're Dad and Scott? And the cats?"

"Dad and Scott are fine. Everything's the same. Weather's hot and muggy at times. It's getting chilly up here, though."

"Is it? I sure can't tell."

Winter had arrived in Bethesda. On Saturday, Mary and I shopped for wool caps, mufflers, socks and sweaters for Ross.

With the help of several nurses, he got into the special wheelchair, bundled from head to toe. With tapes, books and journals, he spent a couple of hours outside in the sun. Even with all his extra clothing and blankets, he shivered. Except for the brief visit to the hotel in October, he had been in the hospital with no activity for nine weeks—a direct result of a bad error in placing the cast on his leg after surgery which resulted in necrosis, leaving a deep hole on the top of his foot.

Another skin graft was scheduled for the following Monday. Since the tendon had been cut, maybe the graft would take. This meant being immobile again for a week before the bandage could be removed.

We resumed the bathing routine, with Ross doing most of the work. This time, he wasn't particular, and often didn't care whether he had a bath or not. I noticed that the strange little spot in the incision line on his leg was still there, unchanged. There seemed to be no point in mentioning it again.

It appeared that Ross would have to remain in the hospital through Thanksgiving. I wasn't sure why. Nothing was going on. I don't think anyone knew what to do with him. No physical therapy or chemotherapy was planned. The ever-present possibility of getting a serious infection in his foot was in everyone's mind.

I stayed with him until the following Saturday evening, when I left NIH in a driving rain. When I called him the next day to see how the skin graft looked, he said the doctors didn't seem pleased. There was no hope that he could come home for Thanksgiving. He had to remain in bed at all times.

Bill flew to Washington on Wednesday, and on Thursday Mary went to NIH to spend the day. In addition to the Thanksgiving dinner provided by organizations in the community, a mother of a former roommate of Ross brought a complete holiday meal for him, Bill, and Mary. She even brought her good china, silver, and crystal.

I drove to Huntsville to be with Scott, and arrived in time for us to have a late Thanksgiving dinner in a restaurant. He took me on a tour of Huntsville, timing his drive so we could see the city at sunset from the top of a mountain. Since so much had transpired in both our lives, we talked continuously, and I was pleased to see how well and happy he seemed to be.

Tuesday, the day after Bill arrived home, we were called and told that Ross could come home for a few days on the following Thursday. Someone would have to return to NIH to travel home with him. I wondered if they were aware of the cost of air fare from Mobile to Washington, and why they couldn't have made this decision one day earlier while Bill was still there.

Bill returned to NIH on Wednesday. At last, Ross came home, almost three months after he left. With Bill beside him, he hobbled slowly on his crutches up the long ramp at the arrival gate, still refusing a wheelchair. He was scheduled to return to NIH a week later so that the surgeons could again look at his foot.

∾

December, 1988

Our house had not been designed for a convalescent. Since we had no downstairs bedroom, we opened a sofa bed in the den and put a real mattress on it. I rented hospital equipment and Sally brought a wheelchair. Bill installed hand grips in the half-bath downstairs.

He became proficient at taking care of Ross's foot—the soaking and dressing changes four times a day. He developed a routine, attending to Ross's foot in the morning before he left for work, at noon when he went home for lunch, on arrival home at 5:30 p.m., and then again at 10:00 at night. It was such a relief for me to have someone share the responsibilities. When I came home from work in the evenings, Ross's friends were usually assisting Bill, and often there was a girl on the bed beside Ross with her head on his pillow.

After only one week at home, Ross and I returned to NIH for an appointment in the Surgery Clinic. When Dr. Cook came to the door of the waiting room to call him, I said, "Ross, mention that funny-looking spot in the incision line. It's still there and it just doesn't look right."

"I'll mention it," he said, as he grabbed his crutches and hopped along the hall.

A few minutes later, Dr. Cook hurried back out into the waiting room. "We're going to have to admit Ross. Something's developed that we have to take care of immediately. We're going to have to go back in...it's to be treated as an emergency...I've scheduled surgery for tomorrow morning."

The magazine I had been scanning dropped from my hands and slipped onto the floor as I sat, dumbstruck. "What? Why? What's wrong?" I asked.

"I've just discovered something which could be very serious.

One of the large sutures we used during surgery has worked its way near the surface—leaving an open avenue for infection directly to the prosthesis," he said.

"What do you mean? What suture?"

"This particular suture is like a heavy shoestring. We used it to tie the muscles to the implant. It goes round and round the muscle. Somehow, the end of it has worked its way out near the surface."

"That's the same spot I've been trying to tell you about for three months. It hasn't just worked its way out. It's been there all the time."

"When I tried to remove it this morning, I discovered it was the end of the suture. These things happen," he said, as he whirled on his heel and walked away.

Not a word had he spoken about what to expect or what the surgery would entail. No reassurance was offered that this would be easily corrected or that I shouldn't worry. No time was given for further questions. My rebuttal of his statement that the suture had worked its way out near the surface had shocked and angered him, but he could hardly deny it since I had asked about the funny-looking spot so many times. I surmised that he couldn't think of a way to blame me for it.

We had flown up for this short appointment and had planned to go home the following day. Now, Ross had to be admitted, returned to surgery, and only God knew what was going to be done this time, or how long he would have to stay.

Ross's eyes looked weary as he slowly hobbled toward me. He pressed his lips together tightly. When we reached the elevator, he struggled into the car, and we started moving down. He leaned his back against the wall, closed his eyes, and remained silent. Perspiration outlined his upper lip.

When we reached the main lobby, I asked, "Would you like me to get a wheelchair?"

He shook his head.

"Go on up to thirteen, Ross. I'll get you admitted."

"You can't do that. I have to sign the papers," he said with trembling lips.

"They'll have to take the papers up to you," I said.

He worked his way slowly through the gallery to the elevator of the hospital wing. The clerk in the admitting office said she would be glad to take the consent forms to him. She had admitted him so many times before.

Surgery was scheduled for 8:00 Saturday morning. Dr. Malawer was called and arranged to be there. I canceled our hotel reservation and moved our luggage to the 13th floor.

Early the next morning, an anesthesiologist visited Ross in his room. Since he had never met Ross before, he introduced himself and told us he couldn't really discuss his case because he hadn't seen Ross's record. No one knew where the file was.

"Is it because it's Saturday?" I asked.

"Shouldn't be," he said. "But nobody seems to know where it is. I'll ask Dr. Cook if he has it."

After he left, I leaned against the door frame and watched as he talked to Dr. Cook near the nurses' station. They spoke to a nurse and she hurried to a phone. Obviously, Dr. Cook was telling the anesthesiologist that he didn't have the file.

Suddenly, Dr. Cook whirled and came tromping along the hall toward Ross's room. In a louder than necessary voice, he called to me, "Are you responsible for this? Do you have Ross's record? Have you retained a lawyer?"

Several nurses nearby looked aghast.

"I don't know what you're talking about," I said.

His anger spent, he spun around and walked back behind the nurses' station. Ross had heard him, and I thought, What a great way to go to surgery, with one of your surgeons acting like an ogre. Immediately, I thought of many things I wished I had said to him. I wondered how in the world he thought I could have gotten the record during the night, even if the thought of a lawsuit had entered my mind.

With wide-stretched eyelids, the head nurse apologized to me for the doctor's behavior. The hall gossip machine switched on. Thank God, Dr. Malawer would operate. I wished that Dr. Cook could have been barred from entering the surgery theater.

Dr. Malawer had Ross's file. I was sorry I didn't think of that possibility. Somebody should have thought of it.

Ross was placed on the gurney, and I rode down in the

elevator with him to the surgery floor. At the big double doors, I kissed him on his forehead. No one told me what to expect or how long he would be in surgery. I supposed they didn't know.

When I rode the elevator to the cafeteria, the building seemed deserted on this early Saturday morning. I tried to imagine how Ross might feel after this operation. If the suture went around the muscle, would it have to be re-routed so the end would be tucked safely away? How much would the muscles be moved around? Would the nerves and blood vessels be involved? Would the pain be as bad as before? The agony he suffered was caused by removal of bone, rearrangement of muscles, nerves and blood vessels, and the incomprehensible pressure on the top of his foot where the cast had been put on improperly.

With a heavy feeling of dread, I left the cafeteria. As I walked along the hall, I met one of the oncologists I had known since 1982. A quiet, kind and humble man, he usually dressed in sports clothes with rarely a cover-up of the traditional white jacket. His eyes twinkled when he smiled.

"Good morning, Mrs. Phelps," he said. "What are you doing here? I thought Ross was discharged."

"He was, but he's back again," I said, while staring at the floor.

"What's the matter?" he asked. "I remember six years ago when you and Ross were here, you kept your chin up and had a nice smile. Is there something wrong? Why is Ross admitted?"

When I told him of the problem, I confessed that I felt it was gross negligence on the part of whoever closed after surgery and left the end of the suture so near the surface. I expressed my feeling about the incompetence of whoever put the cast on.

"I'm so sorry, Mrs. Phelps. You must talk to the surgeons and let them know how you feel. Talk to Dr. Cook."

"I can't talk to Dr. Cook."

"Why not?"

"Because he is...he's inconsiderate, arrogant...he's a pompous ass! I'm sorry...I'm so exasperated with this whole thing," I whispered.

"No apology needed. I've often had similar thoughts about

him myself—and worse," he said. "Let me know if I can do anything."

As I had been instructed, I returned to the surgery waiting room, where I sat for three hours. When I went to the 13th floor to ask a nurse to call surgery, I learned that Ross had already been returned to his room by the back elevator. No one came to the waiting room to tell me it was finished or what had happened.

Ross slept as I sat beside his bed wondering how he could travel still another painful road. For most of the afternoon, his eyes were closed. He had never stopped taking pain medication from the original surgery, and received even more through the IV connected to the Port-A-Cath. He didn't complain that evening or during the night.

The next day, I figured out why. He had no feeling in that portion of his leg. There had been no new pain because numbness still remained from the original surgery three months ago. He was to remain in bed indefinitely.

No one ever told me what the surgery entailed. It may have been a simple procedure, but I never knew. I never saw Dr. Cook again to ask. I never looked for him and knew he was avoiding me. That was all right with me. He must have felt some embarrassment, and, it is to be hoped, a little remorse.

Four days after his operation, I left Ross alone and returned to Mobile to get back to work. He picked up where he left off before the surgery. He watched movies on the VCR, staff visited him, and other patients' caregivers brought him things from the newsstand and cafeteria.

He began drawing cartoons, using "Calvin" of comic book fame as his guide. He placed Calvin in situations similar to the patients in the hall. In one sketch, Calvin was a "mad scientist," mixing chemotherapy—an experimental protocol especially designed for a certain doctor which contained iguana blood and squid eyeballs. Sometimes wicked-looking Calvin held a huge needle, ready to place into a nurse's derriere. Calvin complained about the food, about wanting to be released from his prison, and of his loneliness. In some scenes, Calvin was risque or angry; in another, he longingly held a piece of mistletoe over his head. In one drawing, he was crying.

Drawing had always been effortless for Ross; however, I had never known him to draw cartoons. The souvenir box at home had many of Scott's creations of funny characters speaking witty lines, but Ross's drawings were usually more serious.

Even before he started kindergarten, Ross could draw remarkably well, with good perspective and attention to details. When he was five years old, while sitting in the back seat of the car on a trip to the Gulf, he quietly created the interior of a museum, with people looking up at a huge dinosaur skeleton. The bones and joints of the skeleton were clearly delineated. His museum visitors were well defined, not "stick people," and included details in their clothing.

Another one of his very early works revealed not only artistic talent but his budding personality as well. He drew a construction site with a building in progress. All his workmen were identified as either his dad, Scott, uncles, or male cousins. They each had a tool in their hands; some were standing on scaffolding and others were on ladders. On the ground, with hands on hips, stood the overseer of the job. He wore a hardhat and was identified as "Ross."

Another interesting drawing in my collection was his final art project when he was a senior in high school: A pen and ink drawing of an eagle's claw.

He gave some drawings to Mark Daullary who was back on the hall, going downhill every day. His parents often stopped to say hello to Ross, but Mark could no longer leave his bed.

Finally, on December 21st, Ross received permission to come home. Mary got him out of the hospital, to the airport, and accompanied him to Mobile.

He set up residence again in the den, and in the morning, when I checked on him, I found his wastebasket full of used tissues. I didn't know if his tears came from sadness or from joy.

31

Jean, Russell, and Tosh brought us the biggest Christmas tree we had ever had. They had spotted it at a farm and had enlisted their friends to help deliver it to us.

Bill made the annual Christmas trip to Troy to visit his mother and sister, then drove the very long trek to Huntsville to get Scott. Scott's car had made its final highway trip. When they returned to Mobile on Friday evening, our family was together for the first time in many months.

During the morning of Christmas Eve Day, a nurse called from NIH to tell Ross that Mark Daullary had died. He had left the hospital the same day Ross did and had died in his home town.

"He was a real good kid!" Ross said. He slammed his fist down on the kitchen counter. With tears brimming, he turned to me and repeated softly, "He was a really good kid."

I put my arms around him and said, "I know how you felt about Mark. He loved you, Ross."

"The Daullarys probably asked the nurse to let me know since it's against the rules for them to tell people when someone dies."

He fastened his crutch on his prosthesis, went outside to his hammock, and lay there watching the sky.

∾

Company started arriving. The Riordas came from New Orleans and Dorothy decorated our tree—a detail we had left undone. Jean and her family, Joe and Vilma, friends and neighbors dropped in. Scott and Mary took charge of the traditional fudge-making ritual with a kitchen full of people.

After everyone left, Ross and I were in the living room when he said, "I'd like to go to the midnight service at church but I can't. I'm too tired."

"Don't worry about it. We'll skip this year. I'm bushed, too."

"But I really would like to go."

"Rest for awhile, and see if you can take a nap. If you feel better, we'll go."

I stretched out on another sofa, turned out all the lights except those on the Christmas tree, and fell asleep. Scott slipped in and made funny pictures of us.

In a little while, we woke. "Can we still go?" Ross asked. "I can't sit in the pew. My leg has to stick straight out."

Stretching, yawning, and rubbing my eyes, I said, "I'll ask for a couple of folding chairs and put them in the back."

"And I can't go up for communion."

"Don't worry about it. You don't have to. The elders will bring it to you," I mumbled.

"No, I don't want that."

"Then just skip it, Ross. You don't have to take communion. There's no church law that says you have to."

"I don't care if there's a law or not. If I'm going to attend anything, I want to participate. Let's go."

The rest of the family had gone out or up to bed when we left for church. Over Ross's objections, I parked the car in the reserved handicapped space. When we entered the building, an usher placed two chairs in the back behind the pews. I propped the crutches up in the corner.

The service, as usual, was moving and beautiful in the candle-lit sanctuary. We joined in singing the old favorite carols. When the time came for communion, ushers stood by each row of pews, directing people to the altar, one group at a time. As the ushers moved closer to the back, Ross reached for his crutches.

When our turn came, I walked ahead of him to the altar and waited. He came down the aisle alone. When we finished the sacraments with others at the table, we returned to our seats and the service soon ended.

An usher held a door open, and we were among the first outside into the cool midnight air. As we stood, greeting friends as they left the sanctuary, I noticed many tears and thought it was the sentimentality of the occasion and service. Then, it dawned on me. Ross had brought forth the emotion. Again, I had forgotten how people might react when they saw him. I wondered if our presence there on this holy night intruded into other people's lives of order and serenity—their peace on earth.

Later, after pondering, wondering and worrying about it, I concluded that many hearts were already saddened by their own personal memories over the years. Ross had only brought forth tears that were already there. Still, we might have been thoughtlessly selfish in wanting to be there, among our friends.

Perhaps this is how it begins when one decides to become a recluse.

The next day, we had an early Christmas dinner because Mary had to fly back to Washington. On Monday Bill returned to his office, and Scott left for Huntsville with friends who had come home for the holiday.

After everyone had gone and the house was quiet, Ross said, "Don't you think this has been the best Christmas ever?"

The grief, suffering, and fear of the past six months flashed through my mind as I gazed out the window.

"It's been a good Christmas...yes, it has."

On Thursday after Christmas when I came home from work, Ross called me into the living room. He sat on the sofa with the crutches nearby. "I want you to see something," he said, as he rose and stood, placing his right foot down on the floor.

"Wonderful, Ross! Are you putting any weight on it?"

"That's not all. Watch."

With great concentration and deliberation, he moved his right foot forward a few inches, then his left foot, and then his right one again.

"All right! Look at you! Come see, Bill! That's wonderful!"

He stood proudly with his shoulders back and had a bright smile on his face before he sat back down.

He didn't try it again until the next day when Paul came to see him. The two of them were about finished with their visit when I got home.

"Ross, have you told Paul what you can do?" I asked.

"Not yet," he said.

"Show him. He deserves to share the good news."

He stood, straightened his shoulders and, taking a deep breath, walked several small steps. He bowed to Paul's applause before returning to the sofa.

He couldn't bend his knee, but he had good balance. He really could walk. Although the crutches were always near at hand, he practiced a little every day, and began to believe in the miracle.

He savored his time at home to the fullest. He was scheduled to return to NIH on January 4th for CT scans and an appointment with a plastic surgeon.

32

January, 1989

We left on the first Wednesday of the new year. Although we had pleasant weather in Mobile, the Washington area had freezing rain, so again, Ross refused to fly into National Airport.

Huddling close together against the terminal building at Dulles, we shivered while watching for the NIH shuttle. We had been misdirected to our bus stop, and, when the van finally arrived, we and our luggage were a long walk away.

When we spotted the bus, Ross decided to try to carry the backpack. He was using his crutches, and when I tried to assist him in placing the heavy bundle across his back, I managed to catch him as he fell backward.

The sad, pained expression on his face when he realized he couldn't do it revealed more than the disappointment of knowing he couldn't help me. The backpacking trip had still been a hope for the future. He began to acknowledge that he was a long way from being strong enough to even think about it.

We went directly to the out-patient clinic, where his blood was drawn for the usual checks. Several patients he knew from 1982 were also in the clinic that day. We saw John Talbert, who was there for his yearly check-up. John was a young teenager when we first met him, and now he was a handsome, healthy-looking young man. He had experienced no problems with the Ewing's sarcoma which was found in his rib. Now a senior in college, he was into strenuous cross-country bicycling. His mother, Elise, still had the pretty smile.

After visiting the 13th floor to say hello to Ross's friends, we checked into the Marriott for our three-night stay. The next morning, we woke to a snow-covered landscape, and proceeded to the clinic for the appointment with the plastic surgeon. I sat in the waiting room while Ross was being examined.

In a few minutes, he came out and said, "Guess what, Mom. I'm going to be admitted."

"Oh no, don't tell me that! What for this time?"

"The doctor says there's another tendon that can be cut, and after that, he wants to try another skin graft."

Skin graft meant another week in bed.

"You don't have to stay, Mom. They're not going to put me to sleep. It's going to be done under local."

"I don't know what to do, Ross. I told the staff I'd be back to work on Monday."

"Plan to go on home. It's okay."

After he was admitted on Sunday, I caught the shuttle to National Airport and returned home. On Monday, the surgeons clipped the tendon, applied another graft, and ordered another week of immobility.

There was nothing more to say. He listened to his meditation tapes, read what he could, and watched every movie in the library, plus some the recreation staff brought from their homes.

The following Sunday, he called home to say that the doctors had removed the bandage and the graft looked good. Our hopes began to rise. Monday's report was also good. Tuesday, the report was questionable. This meant remaining in bed for another week until it was admitted that the procedure had failed again. It was two weeks later before he was told he could go home, three weeks after he had arrived.

Mary accompanied him home. In addition to filling a needed role for us, she was taking a break from her stressful life in Virginia.

When I looked at Ross's foot, I could see that the hole on the top hadn't changed, so Bill again began his routine of changing dressings four times a day.

Ross decided he wasn't going to worry about his foot any longer, and was going to get on with his life. He announced he was ready to move upstairs into his own room and his own bed for the first time in four months. He was going to take a bath—a real bath in the shower.

Bill helped him to place his foot in a plastic bag and step into the shower. Had he been stronger, he would have stayed an hour under the tingling water. Although he had been without a full bath for a long time, he had done well with the lavatory scrub downstairs. His hair had grown back again, and I helped him every day with shampoos. These simple things would be etched in his mind forever.

He wanted to figure out some way to drive his car, which had remained in the driveway since his surgery in September. In 1986, I gave up trying to share a vehicle with him, and bought him a car. He'd selected the smallest, least expensive car in the Honda line, which turned out to be a two-seater. I wasn't in favor of this, but was reminded that the only restrictions I had placed on his selection were that it had to fit my budget plans and have automatic transmission.

On Saturday, I drove him to a specialty shop, where we discussed an adaptor for the brake and accelerator. The left foot would have to do all the work.

I recalled the day I first rode with him after his arm amputation while he was behind the wheel. A daring 18-year old, proving he could adapt to the circumstances, he took chances he never would have risked when he'd had two hands. At that time, I wondered if there wasn't some law on the books which forbade driving with your left knee. Now, over six years later, a mature 24-year-old man wanted to be safe.

We returned home from the shop and he thought about it. Using the left foot for both gas pedal and brake didn't seem as safe as he would like. He went out to his car and sat awhile.

A few days later, he came to me and said, "Mom, I'm going for a drive. I want to try something."

At last, I had learned to keep my mouth shut.

In a few minutes he was back, still pondering. "I've decided not to have an adaptor put on. As my leg gets stronger, I can rest it on the gas pedal and use my left foot on the brake. I think it'll work."

"You tried it already?"

"Just around the block. My leg hurts too much and it's too weak, but I think it's the safest way."

Maybe, I thought, if he used the left foot for the brake, he wouldn't be steering the car with his left knee. This turned out not to be true. He still managed to lift his knee to the steering wheel when he needed to use his right hand for something else.

February, 1989

In his telephone calls to NIH, Ross learned that too much time had elapsed for him to continue participating in the study. It appeared that no one knew the best course of action to take.

His hair, dark brown with a few red highlights, had grown back completely and needed a trim. He had regained most of his weight and was feeling pretty well. Except for pain in his leg, for which he still took medication, and the body cramps when his magnesium was too low, he seemed to be as normal as he had been in years.

When he was in Mexico in 1987, he had brought back a string hammock, so, on warm days, he spent hours in the back yard, reading, listening to tapes, or just watching the clouds, birds, and airplanes go by. He was glad to be home, but the tension of not knowing what would be coming next was always present.

Ross had never been seriously hooked on television. Since he had watched it so much while in the hospital, he didn't care to turn it on. He was thoroughly bored. While day-dreaming, he was obviously again planning how to improve the looks of our yard and patio. He mentioned again how nice it would be to have a fountain and a fish pond.

"Then let's start planning one," I said. "Decide where you want it, draw it out on paper, and find out the cost involved."

"I thought you said Dad didn't want it out here."

"Suppose we just don't mention it. If we make a big mess, we can always put it back like it was." I placed a small table by the hammock for his paper, pencils, and calculator.

Paul visited him often and could be found outside sitting in a chair near the hammock. I never knew what they talked about and wondered if Ross was truly expressing his fears and questions to Paul. One day, when walking with Paul to his car, I asked, "Do you think Ross realizes the gravity of his situation?"

"When one asks the kind of questions Ross does, I can certainly assume that he understands. For instance, 'Do you think people are aware of the presence of God at the moment of death?' That's a profound question, especially coming from someone as young as he is."

When Ross called NIH again to find out what, if anything, was being discussed about his case, he got the impression that it was up to him to make the decision about continuing chemotherapy. I suggested that we talk to Dr. Clarkson, and we made the appointment. Dr. Clarkson was sympathetic to both sides of the dilemma, but also felt that Ross shouldn't have the burden of making the decision. He suggested that Ross put the question back on the NIH oncologists' shoulders.

Since he had to return to NIH the following week for an appointment in the surgery clinic, he called and asked for a conference with the oncologists. We made a list of our questions and Ross started packing—loading up clothes, books, tapes and stationery.

"We're only going to be there one day, Ross. I'm not lugging all this stuff up there," I said.

"Surely you know by now to expect the unexpected. I'm taking no chances. They may decide to admit me," he insisted.

We met with Dr. Horowitz and Dr. Smith, taking turns with our list of questions. Since Ross no longer fit the protocol, what would happen? The oncologist in charge of the protocol had seemed distant, and I didn't know who would be following his case. They may have had definite plans for Ross but were not very good in articulating that fact to us.

The decision was made that Ifosfamide would be continued as soon as the surgeons released him. The VP 16 would be dropped. The risks to his foot and leg versus the possible benefits were too great to continue the VP 16.

I asked if consideration was given to stopping treatment altogether, since so much time had passed and we still didn't know when he could get started. Their conclusion was the same as before: If there were any malignant cells in Ross's body, the Ifosfamide could be effective in eliminating them. If no treatment was given, and a metastasis occurred, the Ifosfamide would not be as effective.

Ross discussed his long-range plans for study and asked about traveling in Third World countries. Dr. Horowitz urged him to keep his plans, and by the time he was ready to start this venture, he should be able to travel with little difficulty.

He looked up Andy Tartler, who was now the Executive Director of a new project for Special Love, a cancer support group. The project—development of a place for out-patient pediatric patients and their families to stay when at NIH—would be located on property directly across the street from the hospital in a picturesque landscape.

Ross asked Andy if there was any way he could stay in Bethesda and get a job as his assistant. Andy wanted to hire him, but there was no funding. The building, known as The Children's Inn, was being designed and constructed through the efforts of benefactors, and all funds would necessarily have to go to the development.

When we returned to the hotel, I said, "Can you believe it? We're actually going to get to go home tomorrow. Nobody said anything about admitting you."

"Don't be too sure, Mom. It's still early. Let's don't answer the phone if it rings."

We escaped home the following day, lugging the heavy backpack. At least a decision had been made. Treatment would begin when and if the surgeons gave up.

∾

March, 1989

Paul knew of Ross's restlessness and desire to try to work part time while in treatment. He arranged an appointment for him in the International Department of his bank. From there, Ross visited with another family friend who routed him to other departments, where one kind lady made an appointment for him at a shipping company downtown.

He was very excited about his interviews. His resume was carefully prepared and he put on his best suit and tie. He had been able to wear only his old sneakers, loosely tied over the right foot, so we shopped for a pair of soft, black sport shoes. Confidently, he drove himself downtown. He received such courtesy and interest that when he returned home, he stood a little taller.

"I think they liked me," he beamed.

"Why wouldn't they?"

"I didn't figure I'd pass their 'image test'."

"You present a very good image. Anyone would be glad to have you."

"It may be hard for me to find a job."

He couldn't make a commitment to anything, because coming up the following week were bone scan, CT scans, and appointments in the surgery clinic of NIH. This time he wanted to drive. He was fed up with airports, airplanes, and shuttles. Natalie Kaiser, James Hutchins' girlfriend, was on spring break from school, and he asked her to drive up with him. James was in Mexico on the first leg of the long-awaited trip.

Natalie, a hard-working, brilliant student was dedicated to her goal of working with the dispossessed around the world. She dressed conservatively, wore no makeup, and her long light brown hair fell past her shoulders. With her ever-present smile, she promised she would do all the driving.

They spent one night with Jo Bonner, who had recently returned to the Congressional office where he would soon become Chief of Staff. While Ross was at NIH, Natalie rode the metro to various appointments she had made, checking out possibilities of positions with service organizations throughout the world.

Ross's tests were clear except for the spot on his lung which still appeared unchanged. He wasn't dismissed by the surgeons—the hole in his foot was still there.

When he returned home on Friday, the waiting hung heavily on him. He still couldn't make plans.

We had discussed the fountain and fish pond many times, and he had drawn a rough sketch of what he wanted. He made photographs of the site and purchased a booklet on the care of pond fish. We had looked at statuary places but found nothing that interested either of us.

On the Saturday evening before Easter, we were sitting on the patio discussing what we had in mind about the pond. The more we talked, the bigger the pond grew in Ross's mind. He wanted a moving stream from one section of the patio to the other, with a little bridge across it for the cats to use.

"Ross, we're miles apart. What I see is just a small pond, something for the water from the fountain to fall into. We can put a few fish in it and listen to the sound of the water. It's the music of the waterfall that I'm interested in."

"But it would look so nice out here, Mom. It wouldn't be any harder to build."

I had already spoken with a man who worked with concrete and stone about what I thought Ross had in mind, and even for a small area his charge was prohibitive. We would have to do it ourselves. "You can't help with the digging and I know I can't dig a large area. Be realistic," I said.

"I think I can help. Maybe I can. Let's get started."

"When? Now? At this hour? No way. Tomorrow is Easter and we're going to Lucedale. Wait until the first of the week."

"Let's just see how hard it is to dig."

"Give me a break, Ross. Let's don't get into it at this late hour."

"Let's just see if the ground is hard. It'll only take a little while."

If the neighbors had seen us at midnight, digging in our yard, they might have called the police. I loosened the dirt with the shovel, and Ross, using a small spade in his right hand, picked up the soil. When I hit a tree root, he used a hatchet on it, bending down on his left knee and keeping his right leg straight out. We made great headway.

The next morning, Bill glanced at the pile of dirt, but said nothing. We went to the Easter gathering at Jean's and joined in the fishing rodeo. Ross was extremely tired, and so was I.

When we returned home, Sunday notwithstanding, we began again. We argued about the depth, the length, and the width. Finally, exhaustion took over and he agreed we could stop, except that the hole had to be made deeper at one end.

During the next few days, we looked for stones. We purchased the biggest part of the investment—the pump. We visited a supply company and bought some pieces of slate Ross had said we needed for the fountain. Our friends and neighbors contributed stones from their yards. On automobile trips when our children were small, we had collected rocks from every state we passed through. They were half buried in our yard now, but we dug them up and added them to the growing pile.

Finally, although Ross wasn't completely satisfied with the size, we stopped digging. It had reached about ten feet in length. The sides curved, the width varying from five feet to two feet. The depth at one end was only one foot, but it slanted to three feet at the fountain site.

Taking out the instruction book, Ross said we needed lots of old magazines and catalogues. We gathered them from around the house and placed them side by side all over the bottom of the hole, covering the soil and any tree roots we had missed. Then we spread heavy polyethylene over the magazines. We anchored it along the edges with heavy rocks, and trimmed the excess plastic all around the area, leaving the ends to be buried under the dirt. At last, it was ready to add the water.

Ross arranged and rearranged the rocks to create the effect he wanted. He placed the sheets of slate in tiers, extending them over the water so that, when the stream fell from the rocks, an echo chamber would be formed.

We turned the switch on. At last, after so many years, he had his fountain.

The next morning, we were pleasantly surprised to see the water was still there. Both of us went to work rearranging rocks, adjusting the fountain tubes, and picking up the mess we had made. Although we hadn't done a perfect job, we were pleased with the outcome.

We designed flower beds around the pond, and visited nurseries to buy begonias and impatiens. Ross could hardly wait to let the water settle so he could put goldfish in it. He found some minnows in a stream on Spring Hill College's campus.

At the end of three weeks, we stepped back and looked. The little goldfish seemed to be at home in their new environment. While it didn't look professionally built—plastic showing in several places—we thought it was beautiful. To complete the picture in my mind, I decided to pursue getting a swing placed near the pond.

Lewis Mayson put heavy posts in the ground next to the patio and Joe Croom brought a swing and hung it. It was such a pleasant place to be. We should have done it years ago.

The raccoons discovered the pond, and during the night they often rearranged the rocks and took the fountain apart. Once we found the tubing for the pump on the other side of the house. As the weather got warmer, Ross was convinced the raccoons were doing belly dives and swimming laps in the little pond. He could hear them from his window, playing and splashing during the night. As far as we know, they never caught a fish, and soon became disenchanted with the novelty. The birds and cats seemed to welcome a place to drink water.

The pond and fountain would prove to be a source of pleasure and comfort in the months to come.

33

April, 1989

The waiting was soon to be over. Dr. Smith called and asked Ross to come back for another chest X-ray and conference. It was possible that chemotherapy could begin soon.

He flew to Washington alone and caught the shuttle to NIH. After he had a chest X-ray, he was told that the Ifosfamide could be started immediately. He could take the drugs home with him and get the treatment in the Mobile Infirmary.

The amended protocol—only one drug instead of two—was seven months late. When Ross returned to Mobile on April 19, 1989, we went straight from the airport to Dr. Clarkson's office, picked up hospital orders, turned in the drugs, and went to the admissions office of the Mobile Infirmary.

Everything was so different from NIH. When Ross was in the Infirmary six years before, there was a new cancer wing, but, for some reason, he was never placed there. This time, he was in that section. There were no other young patients. Most of them were quite elderly and very, very sick. There appeared to be few nurses—all of them very intent on whatever they were doing. No one looked at us or said hello as we passed the nurses' station.

The private, spacious room was much cleaner and in better

condition that the rooms on the pediatric floor at NIH. It was very quiet compared to what we had been experiencing.

Ross's nurse came in and introduced herself. She wore a white uniform—an oddity for us. She was very precise, professional, and in a great hurry. Later, others came in to check vital signs or to answer his call. Evidently, they were more knowledgeable about chemotherapy than I remembered from before. Dr. Clarkson obviously had given Ross carte blanche on whatever premeds he thought he would need. He told the nurse what he wanted, when he wanted it, and how he wanted it administered. She didn't question him.

It was 10:00 p.m. before the Ifosfamide was started, and Ross asked Bill and me to leave as soon as the nurse came in with the premeds.

Early the next morning, before going to work, I hurried back to the hospital to check on him and leave my phone numbers at the nurses' station. They told me he had complained of nausea but didn't vomit during the night. When I opened his door, his eyes were closed, so I didn't disturb him. Some of the young nurses began to notice and take a special interest in him.

One of Ross's anti-nausea medicines was often referred to as the "memory drug" which, when taken before the chemotherapy, could cause the patient to have no memory of the experience. Ross had tried this drug with some degree of success when he was treated during the previous summer at NIH. The validity of the "memory drug" designation was proven to me when he would call my office and ask me to bring something to him. When I arrived with the requested item, he had no recollection of having called me. He appreciated the antiemetic effect of the drug, but he hated not being able to remember. He had several visitors while in the hospital but could hardly recall who came or when.

The Ifosfamide was given, followed by mesna, for five nights. When I visited him, I took a hanging basket of impatiens and placed it in his room, and when he was discharged, we placed the plant by the fish pond.

Following Ross's release from the hospital, James Hutchins came in from Mexico and spent the weekend with us. Natalie came for dinner on Saturday and they took Ross out to visit friends. James's next trip was to be to Japan. Rebecca Crow had decided to enter graduate school in Arizona the previous fall, and her summer plans would take her to Europe. Natalie was soon to leave for Africa. I tried to tell Ross that someday, he would travel wherever he chose.

The swing, fish pond, fountain, and hammock became his refuge. When he felt like doing nothing else, he put pillows in the swing and lay there, or sat by the pond and watched the fish. He fed them twice daily, and they soon began to cluster at the top of the water when he appeared. When he reached the edge, they squirmed at the surface with their mouths open like baby birds.

May, 1989

Ross was alone and lonely most of the time. He craved for involvement—anything at all to feel that he was participating in something other than illness. He scanned the want ads, circling the hopeful possibilities. He flipped through some of the old college catalogues. He switched the television on for a few minutes, then got up and left the room.

"I've got to find something to do, Mom. I can't stand wasting my life doing nothing."

"I wouldn't say you're doing nothing. Seems to me that what you're doing is very important."

"I'm talking about work, or school, or anything. I don't want to make a career out of being sick. I'm going to look for a part-time job."

Considering that he would be in the hospital for a week every three weeks, and knowing how lousy he felt in between the treatments, I saw this as an impossibility, but said nothing.

"Do you want to try to set up some interviews?" I asked. "There might be a job for you out there. Who knows?"

"I don't know what to do. My hair is about to fall out again and I don't know how people would feel about me coming to work with a scarf on my head. My suits are getting pretty old. I probably couldn't make enough money to buy the clothes I need."

"You need a new suit? Then let's go shopping. Scott told me that Parisian's is having a sale on men's suits—two for the price of one. I let him put a couple on my charge account in the store in Huntsville. If something comes along you want to try, you'll be ready."

"I don't want you to spend that kind of money. I'd like to work and pay for my own."

"There will be plenty of time for that later. Let's at least see what they have."

He selected a dark gray pinstripe and a navy blue suit. He was always opinionated about ties and shirts so he selected these to add to our purchase. He asked, "Mom, do you think you could find some black silk and make me a scarf—one that would look nice with my suits?"

"I don't know about that. I'll see what I can do."

Mary found a good quality silk in Washington, which she sent to us. Sally hemmed it by hand. It would be his "dress-up" scarf. Now he had two, which would ease the laundry problem.

Two weeks after his treatment, his hair was gone again—the third time he had experienced this indignity.

R oss had often said he wanted to continue some of his research and writing, which he had begun in college. Another idea came to me. Maybe he would enjoy a computer. And I could use one in the non-credit writing class I had signed up for at the University of South Alabama.

We had been discussing computers since before Easter and had looked at several brands. In spite of the fact that I used a computer at work, I knew very little about them, so I asked Ross to check everything out, get prices, and make a list of what we needed. After visiting many shops and listening to all the pros and cons, the big day arrived. We became the owners of a computer, monitor, printer, modem, and a mouse. I had no idea what I had purchased.

When the equipment was delivered, Ross was feeling quite ill, but he watched and listened to the man who delivered and installed it. Later, I thought, he would get into it.

In between treatments, his friends continued to take him to the beach or to visit former classmates who lived in nearby cities. But there was only a day or two when he felt pretty good before it was time for the next round.

One year after diagnosis of the tumor in his leg, he had reached only the half-way mark in the chemotherapy treatment.

∾

June, 1989

A few days after he was discharged from the hospital following the sixth round of chemotherapy, he exerted himself to get things packed to attend Camp Rap-A-Hope. Camp was for one week, and I doubted he could stay more than one night.

"Why don't you wait until later in the week when you feel better?" I asked.

"Why? It's not going to make any difference where I am. I'd rather feel bad at camp than at home."

"You're not going to feel up to looking after kids, Ross. Think about the responsibility."

"If I can't be a counselor, I'll be a camper and let somebody look after me."

I didn't hear from him until the following Wednesday when he had to return to town to see Dr. Clarkson. After his appointment, he called and asked me to meet him for lunch.

We sat in a booth in a barbecue restaurant near the interstate ramp. Ross wore his bright red Rap-A-Hope tee shirt and had the silk scarf on his head. His thin face was ashen, damp with perspiration.

"How's your blood work?"

"Pretty bad...real low."

"Are you going to stay home?"

"No. We have doctors at camp."

"I wish there was a hospital."

"Almost is one. We have a 'med-shed' with everything needed. It's only forty-five minutes to the Infirmary."

"What's going on at camp?"

"The usual. But I'm not contributing much. I'm so tired."

"Lots of sick kids?"

"Lots of kids. Only a few are in treatment."

"What are you doing at camp?"

"Laying around in my hammock, mostly. The campers come around to talk. And I walk around a little."

"Ross, please stay home tonight."

"I'm going back, Mom. There's so much work to do up there. We have fifty-three campers this year—fifty-three kids with cancer. My counts should start rising tomorrow and I'll feel better. Anyway, I'd rather be there than home by myself."

He related some of the funny things that had happened at camp and told of the tricks the children had played on the counselors. Ross wasn't the only amputee at camp that year, but he was the only one who had an arm removed. He had told the little campers that a shark got his arm. Some of them believed him.

Friday was the last night of camp and he invited me to visit.

"I'd love to. What time can I come up?" I asked.

"Why don't you leave right after work and have supper with us. I think some other visitors may be there."

In the parking lot of the cafe, I kissed him on the cheek, and watched as he drove up the ramp and out of sight on the interstate. He was right. It was better to be out and among people than to be home alone, even when feeling ill and weak. When driving back to my office, I began to hope that I was learning again to let him go—with peace in my heart.

My drive to camp was through a pretty, wooded area once I left the interstate. The camp, owned by the Deep South Girl

Scouts Council, had been in use for many years. When I drove through the rustic entrance, I entered a different world that could have been hundreds of miles away from home.

The winding, narrow, bumpy dirt road curved through a thicket of pine trees. I passed a stable and saw little children on horses being led around the ring by red-shirted counselors. Cabins were scattered throughout the woods. In front of the main cabin on a large lake, I saw various kinds of water vehicles. Counselors were teaching campers how to paddle or sail. Some little campers seemed to be along just for the ride.

Ross had seen me driving through the woods and soon joined me by the lake. He had a commitment, and just wanted to say hello but would see me later at the dining cabin. He told me he had given up on trying to walk to his various responsibilities and was driving his car from place to place. His cheeks had a little color. He was smiling and almost energetic.

In the early evening, the campers gathered in a circle where they sang to the accompaniment of a guitar played by an Episcopal minister who had been at camp all week. Then we moved to the dining cabin, where I saw several familiar faces of people serving food, helping the campers, and generally assisting in the kitchen. Everyone was a volunteer.

Ross and I went through the cafeteria-style line and sat at a table with some of the campers of his cabin. It was a noisy, boisterous group, laughing and rough-housing. Many of them looked perfectly normal. Others had no hair. Some limped on their prosthetic leg.

After dinner, the farewell program began with comedy routines, giving of awards, and spontaneous speeches. The farewells began in earnest with thanks to so many people. Some of the campers began crying because they didn't want it to be over. There were tears in other eyes as well.

Doctors, nurses, and other medical professionals had volunteered their time and talents to Camp Rap-A-Hope. Several young married couples of various professions used their vacation time to be there and do anything needed.

Members of the Medical Auxiliary who were responsible for

the camp this year drove back and forth each day to their homes in Mobile because there was no room for them to stay at night. Three of the leaders remained, sleeping on cots in the main cabin. As weary as they were, they maintained their warmth and enthusiasm.

"Elaine, we have an extra cot and would love to have you stay the night with us," Lynne said.

"Oh? I'd love to, but I don't think Ross would want me to."

"He won't care. He'd be glad. Why don't you stay? It's late for you to be driving back home alone," Ginny added.

"I don't have anything with me—nothing to sleep in—no toothbrush."

"No problem. We've got lots of tee shirts and plenty of new toothbrushes."

"I would need to call home..."

"Go ahead. There's a phone in the main cabin. Oh yes, I guess we should warn you. The mosquitos are pretty bad. The screens have holes—but we have some repellent."

"Tell her the rest," Lynne said. "We also have mice, but we've gotten used to them. They really don't bother us much."

"Maybe I'd better think about this," I said. "I think Ross would want me to go on home. But thank you. Next time, I'll come prepared."

While driving out through the tunnel of dense woods in the pitch blackness, I recalled that Ross and some friends had almost convinced some of the little campers that there was such a thing as a wood shark that floated through the trees at night. When I reached the main road, a full moon overhead brought relief. I turned on the tape player while reflecting on my visit. None of the volunteers could ever know the impact of what they were doing. Most of the children there couldn't attend a regular camp and had very little pleasure and fun in their lives. Their medical needs were attended to while they were distracted and enjoying being together. The love they received was better than any medicine ever developed.

What a wonderful respite it had been for the parents of the children. Unless one had been through this experience, there would be no way to understand the bombardment of physical and emotional demands which were constantly placed on parents. Yet, all the volunteers were there. They returned year after year. They were special people.

Saturday, Ross arrived home from Camp-Rap-A-Hope and repacked his backpack for his return to NIH. Bone and CT scans, and appointments in the surgery department were already scheduled.

After he flew to Washington on Monday, Mary called. The day had finally arrived when she made the decision to start a new direction in her life. She was moving home.

She arrived Tuesday and Ross returned home on Wednesday. Friday, round number seven of chemotherapy began. The mountaintop was still a long way off.

Mary's lively imagination and cheerful personality kept some kind of action going all the time. She and Ross teased each other, debated the merits of a singer or a movie, and laughed a lot. She threw herself into many outside activities, and couldn't wait to get someone to listen to what she had done, where she had been, and who she had met. In the late evenings, the computer, which had sat catching dust for several weeks, became her refuge. In the 10 years she had been gone, I had forgotten what it was like to have another female at home to talk to. Ross wasn't lonely anymore.

July, 1989

Cycle number eight came around quickly. After Ross reached his room and while waiting for activity to start, two former high school friends dropped by to see him. They looked much the same as I remembered. Although six years had passed since they graduated, they still looked like boys.

In finding out about their lives since high school, I learned they were both in medical school and were soon to leave for their next assignment. One was going to be a psychiatrist, and the other planned to become a surgeon.

I turned my head away and smiled, wondering what it would be like to learn that your surgeon was a boyish-looking man named "Sparky."

∾

While Ross prepared for surgery at NIH in September, 1988, his Aunt Hilda in California began to learn first-hand about the world of cancer. She had been diagnosed with non-Hodgkins lymphoma, which, like so many other conditions that fall under the umbrella of the word "cancer," had many levels and variations. Hilda felt fairly well, so she continued teaching fifth grade in the Orange County Public School system.

She called and suggested that we meet for a long weekend somewhere away from California and Alabama. It would be impossible, I thought. Ross still had miles to go up the treacherous cliffs of treatment, and the end was not yet in sight. Yet, Mary was home. I could consider it.

Near the end of July, I flew to Reno, Nevada, where I met Hilda at the airport. We rented a car and drove to Lake Tahoe. The mountain air, cool and crisp, contrasted agreeably with the heat and humidity in Mobile. The clear blue sky, the icy crystal water in the lake, and the fragrance of the pine trees on the mountainsides made troubles seem far, far away.

Hilda was thoroughly familiar with Dr. Siegel's work as well as Dr. Gerald Jampolsky's and others. She read her devotional books and practiced her meditations several times a day.

One day we went on a raft down the Truckee River, ending the last portion of the trip going through the rapids—a new experience for both of us. Whirling through those rapids with no end in sight paralleled how I visualized my present life. When spinning around and bounding over rocks, with low-hanging limbs at every curve, the only thing to do was hang on. Oars were useless;

all efforts to guide the raft were to no avail. The rushing water moved on, and took everything with it.

On the plane back to Mobile, I reflected on the passing of time. The years had flown by, fluttering too quickly to grasp and hold. How terribly long some painful hours had been; yet, how short the years had become. I wished I had learned many years ago that I could never postpone living, hoping things would be better later. The bad and the good were mixed up together, and there would be no "later" when life would be free of pain.

When I returned home, I learned that everything had gone well without me. When I told of my trip, no one believed we rode the rapids. I couldn't convince my family that Hilda and I were alone in the raft without a guide. I neglected to tell them that others were doing the same thing. When they finally began to accept that it had actually happened, they thought it was wonderfully funny. The image of their mother and aunt going through the rapids was hilarious.

August, 1989

Only four more rounds of chemotherapy remained for Ross, but it seemed to be an eternity. He felt ill most of the time and had no energy. The only thing he did after showering and getting dressed was sit in the swing and watch the fish in the pond. He had been afraid the cats would try to catch them, but they must have been so domesticated they were afraid of the fish. Ross often chuckled while watching a kitten cautiously lean over the edge of the pond to drink, then suddenly jump back when a fish appeared. The flowers around the pond were surviving beautifully.

When he entered the hospital for the next cycle of treatment, Dorothy was in Lucedale visiting Jean, and the two of them came to Mobile that evening. Vilma joined them, and they all went to the hospital to visit Ross. As soon as it was time for the premed to start, he asked us to leave.

We drove to the Wharf House, a little restaurant on Mobile Bay, where we sat on a deck and had dinner. Darkness slowly settled over the gray waters. Boats of all descriptions approached the drawbridge—sailboats with tall masts, powered by subdued motors; shrimp boats with their deep, laboring sound. The four of us lingered over coffee as we talked for a couple of hours. When I returned home, again I remembered how blessed and rich I was to have sisters.

When Ross got out of the hospital, I told him about the Wharf House. A few days later, he was ready to try it, so we drove down for lunch on Saturday. Heavy, moist clouds hovered over the rolling black water as we watched the shrimp boats return for safety. Rain was threatening, but Ross wanted to sit on the deck.

Our suntanned waitress, dressed in shorts, tee shirt and sandals asked, "You folks want to take a chance on the weather?"

"Yes, it's nice out here," Ross said, gazing at the horizon.

"Okay," she said. "I'll move you inside if it starts to rain."

When she left to place our order, thunder rumbled in the distance. Boats lined up, headed under the drawbridge.

"This is great. I haven't seen the water in a long time."

"I hope the rain stays away."

"I'm not worried about it. I don't care if it does rain. I want to be outside. It smells good."

Our waitress brought our shrimp-loaf sandwiches and suggested we move indoors.

"Not yet, Mom. Let's wait."

The girl opened the thin sun umbrella over our table as misty drops began to fall.

Still gazing in the distance, Ross said, "I'm always going to live close to the water. There's something important about looking at the horizon."

"It puts things in perspective—makes you forget your troubles."

"It makes me feel small, which makes my problems small," he said, eyes focused on the far distance.

"It's peaceful for me," I said.

"Right—even in a thunderstorm."

Our soggy sandwiches were delicious, and we didn't get soaked as we sat in the misty stillness with the only sound coming from the chug-a-lug of the shrimp boats moving inward from the bay.

∼

It was time to return to NIH for a CT and bone scan. This time another friend from Spring Hill College drove him, and they stopped in Huntsville and spent the night with Scott. The next night, they camped out in the Blue Ridge Mountains. When they arrived at NIH, Ross met his new Clinical Associate, Dr. Plotsky, another female. So far in his history, except for two weeks in June, 1988, he'd had only one male associate, Dr. Malcolm Smith.

After he finished at NIH, he and his friend left Bethesda and drove to Augusta, Georgia, where they spent the night, then on to Birmingham where they stayed with other college friends.

∼

September, 1989

After another round of treatment in the Mobile Infirmary, a week before his 25th birthday, we tried to interest him in making plans for a special dinner. Again, he selected the Wharf House, and Bill and Mary went with us. We all sat on the deck and watched the moon rise over the water. Mary and Ross walked out a long pier, pausing along the way to look at fish the night fishermen were pulling in.

There were only two more treatments left. Could we possibly hope the end was in sight? When Ross entered the hospital on Friday for his 11th treatment, I decided to visit Scott in Huntsville. During the seven-hour drive there, I practiced strengthening my resolve to keep a grateful heart. In my weekly letters to Scott, I had spoken of this attitude and suggested that he might like to try it. I wrote to him that negative thoughts and expectations were like shaking his fist in God's face. There would be no way God or man could place a gift in a closed fist. He began to pay attention.

During our visit, he told me he was considering moving back home and reentering the University of South Alabama to continue work on his degree. He spoke of some definite goals he wanted to pursue which would require further study.

I was very pleased with his plan, and immediately started thinking, planning, and wondering how it would work out to have all three grown children living back at home at the same time.

∾

October, 1989

I arrived home before Ross was discharged from the hospital. Only one more round of chemotherapy remained, and that one would have to be at NIH. The end really could be seen. But we didn't feel any excitement—we were afraid to get elated.

Ross decided to honor a tentative previous commitment to be a groomsman in the wedding of his high school friend, M. K. Harless, in Georgia. He went for measurements for his formal wear and bought a pair of black shoes—not knowing if he could wear them for the length of time required. One week after being discharged from the hospital, he drove to Wetumpka to spend the night with James Hutchins. From there, he drove to Savannah, where he joined high school friends in their hotel.

When he left, he took his black silk scarf to wear with the formal morning suit. He packed the other scarf for the many parties he was to attend.

When he returned on Monday, Bill asked, "How did you manage getting yourself dressed—all the buttons and everything?"

"There's always somebody to help. I saw a lot of my friends from Mobile," he said.

I said, "I wish I could have seen you in your fancy gear. Did you wear the black scarf? How did you look?"

"I don't know," he said, shaking his head. "I guess I looked all right. As a matter of fact, I looked good...I looked terrific! If you want to know the truth, I looked goofy." He laughed as he spoke; he'd had a good time.

34

On October 19, 1989, he flew to NIH alone for the 12th and final cycle of chemotherapy. The treatment was begun on Friday, and on Monday, he was wheeled down to the X-ray department on the first floor for a CT scan of his chest.

I planned to go to NIH on Wednesday, and while I was there, I wanted another conference. I wanted to know what was being said, or what they thought, now that this ordeal was finished. I didn't make an appointment with anyone, and wondered how difficult it would be to get a conference. In my mind, I tried to formulate the topics I wanted to inquire about, but wasn't even certain what questions remained to be asked. By this time, I had learned that there were no answers.

The chemotherapy treatments were finished; no one had mentioned further surgery. They had given up trying to close the hole on the top of Ross's foot, which erased the possibility of physical therapy. After one whole year, his foot remained the same in spite of clipped tendons and numerous skin grafts. There seemed to be nothing left to talk about.

When I arrived in Ross's room, he was in the shower and I called to him to let him know I had arrived. As I walked toward the nurses' station, a dark-haired woman carrying a stack of records walked hurriedly toward me. She wore slacks and a white hospital coat, a stethoscope hanging around her neck.

"Are you Mrs. Phelps?" she called. "Ross said you should be here by noon. I'm Dr. Plotsky. Let's talk a minute."

Except for greeting her, I remained silent.

"We've had to repeat Ross's CT scan today. The one he had Monday showed a tiny spot in his lung." She spoke very rapidly, as if she wanted to get it over with.

Like a stunned parrot, I said, "You've repeated it today?"

"Yes, it's still there."

"What does it mean?" I asked.

"Well, for one thing, we know it wasn't a flaw in the film. I must assure you, it's a very tiny spot which could be caused by any number of things. Try not to worry about it."

"Is it the same spot he had before?"

"No, it's not in the same location."

"What happens next?"

"Nothing. We'll just have to wait and watch. He'll get his bone scan tomorrow and repeat the CT scan in a month."

Feeling a very heavy weight descend, I asked, "Can I possibly talk to Dr. Horowitz?"

"Certainly. I'll call him right now. He's in the clinic."

Within minutes, Dr. Horowitz came along the hall. We returned to Ross's room. The water was still running in the shower, and the door was closed.

Dr. Horowitz and I sat on the built-in caregiver's bed while he went over the report, saying essentially the same thing Dr. Plotsky had stated: We would have to wait and watch.

Although Dr. Horowitz had many demands on his time, he seemed relaxed as we spoke. He took the time to go over many aspects of Ross's case. He spoke of the uniqueness of the development and possible progression of the disease. He didn't verbalize anything bright in his future, but somehow I got the impression that he thought Ross was going to be all right.

Dr. Horowitz spoke firmly, yet gently to me, in a personable way, leaving me with a good feeling about him and his interest in Ross. I recalled all the other times he had taken the time to talk to me in words I could understand, even though they weren't what

I wanted to hear. As he left the room, I felt warm and secure—he spoke of Ross as if he belonged to him.

When Ross finally came out of the bathroom, he asked, "Have you heard the news?"

"Yes, they told me. I've spoken to Dr. Plotsky and Dr. Horowitz."

"What did they tell you?"

"The same thing they told you, I'm sure. We'll just have to wait and watch. I'm not upset, Ross. Are you?"

"I'm disappointed."

"I know. So am I, but let's try to put it out of our minds for now. Remember all the false alarms we've had before. Maybe this is just another."

We finished his packing and headed for the elevator. We didn't talk, or even look at each other, while waiting for elevator to reach our floor. When we got on, I stepped to the rear of the car and leaned back against the wall. As we were moving down, a pall of sadness enveloped me. I felt so sorry for Ross, for myself, and for Bill. I debated whether to call Bill with the news or wait until we got home. But when I examined my motive for wanting to call him at that time, I recognized it was my need for comfort, for support. And I knew from past experience that Bill was unable to offer that. He, too, was doing the best he could. Since he never talked about his pain to anyone, I saw no reason to tell him now. Besides, it might be nothing. And even if there was something there, nothing would be done about it any time soon. I didn't want to talk about it with anyone. Ross didn't either.

Before I had left Mobile, I had learned there wasn't a single hotel room to be found in Bethesda or in the neighboring areas. Jo Bonner had volunteered to let us stay in his apartment in Arlington, Virginia, so we got a cab and traveled there.

His apartment seemed like luxury compared to our usual hotel room. Homemade chicken soup awaited Ross, and the refrigerator was stocked with all kinds of good food. Jo stayed with a friend, and, early the next morning, he picked us up and drove us to a metro station on Capitol Hill.

We returned to NIH for a bone scan. The dye injection was at 9:00, and the scan was to be done at noon. As I waited for Ross, I walked the old familiar grounds, wondering how long it would be, if ever, that I would return. I hoped and prayed I would never have to; yet I had a feeling of melancholy at the prospect of saying goodbye forever.

While wandering around outside the building, I saw other caregivers taking a few minutes break from the 13th floor. Their faces were tired, grim, and aged. After crossing the street in front of the Clinic Center, I saw that construction was already under way on The Children's Inn, the Special Love facility on campus. It had been dubbed "Pizzo's Palace" in honor of Dr. Pizzo and his wife, who were prime movers in getting the facility started. How great it would be to have a place so close to the hospital and doctors.

Caregivers were usually nervous about leaving their young patients in the hospital, even for a short time. The children were frightened when they knew their mothers weren't in the building. Sometimes even the older children were afraid.

Actually, age had nothing to do with it. A roommate Ross once had while on the 12th floor was a man who appeared to be between 40 and 50. It was hard to tell. He had a tough, swarthy appearance, and I envisioned him as a dock-worker or a seaman because he had tatoos all over his arms. He was a quiet, non-communicative roommate who never had a visitor when Ross was in the room with him. About the only exchange I could establish with him was a morning greeting when I entered, or a "good-night" when I left the room.

One day, when I was gathering Ross's things to get ready for discharge, I tried again to engage him in conversation.

"I hope you'll be able to get out of here soon. I know it's tough to be stuck here for so long."

"I can leave anytime I want to," he said, a bit defensively.

"Oh? Well, that's great! Are you getting a pass for the weekend, or are you being discharged?"

"Neither. I don't have any place to go. I don't have anyone to take care of me."

He then told me that shortly after one of his chemotherapy treatments, he had suffered a near fatal heart attack. Quietly, he said, "I'm scared. This place is my lifeline."

This monstrous disease can make cowards of us all.

I sat on a bench near the Clinic Center and watched the traffic and pedestrians. When I strolled back to the front entrance under the porte cochere, I felt the chill wind that whipped through the area. I walked toward the elevator, stopping at my favorite piece of sculpture to study the kneeling, hooded figure with hands cupped to receive the healing water. I took a notepad from my purse and tried to do a quick sketch of the figure. Perhaps someday I would find the time to paint it.

When I arrived in the clinic on the 13th floor, again I stood and looked out the window, remembering when I first saw the same scene seven years before in 1982. The view now, very much the same as then, prompted me to wonder how much, if any, I had changed in my ability to see and accept.

Thinking of all the unexpected, surprising "gifts" which came Ross's way during the past seven years, I wondered if the whole experience could be considered a gift—one to be grateful for. No. At least, not yet—too many painful memories; scars too deep. But I didn't want to be bitter. I didn't want to become hard and cynical. I searched for gratitude within me.

Ross's life had been strangely enriched by this experience. He had learned so much—how to live...how to love and receive love...how to get the most out of every day. He loves life, *in spite of*. I would try to hold on to that and be grateful.

The late afternoon sun produced a kaleidoscope of color on the landscape beyond the window. Ross walked up and joined me, standing silently, gazing into the distance. After a few minutes of meditative quiet before the panorama, I asked, "All finished? Can we leave now?"

"Not yet. I'm going on the hall to visit someone."

"Who? Anyone I know?"

"No. I don't know who it is yet. All I know is that it's a girl who just had her leg amputated. Wait for me here. Okay?" He turned away. I watched as he walked slowly, yet confidently, along the corridor toward the hospital wing.

The work day, drawing to a close, slowed the activity in the waiting room. The staff began tidying their work areas, but the ever-constant phone-ringing had not abated.

After waiting about 30 minutes, I saw Dr. Plotsky and asked, "If there's a problem showing on the CT scan, won't it show up on the bone scan done today?"

"Possibly. Yes, it most likely will if it's large enough."

Ross approached as we were talking and asked the doctor if she had seen the results of the bone scan.

"No, but I'll go right now, Ross. Wait here," she said as she headed for the elevator.

A little later she returned with a big smile on her face. "Good news, Ross! I asked the technicians, and they said it was an utterly boring scan. Not a single thing on it!"

"What now? Does it really mean anything?" Ross asked.

She put her arm around him and said, "Try not to worry. Something is on the CT. We'll take another look next month."

Ross had been asked to visit another patient who was facing amputation, but he could not. He was too weak and tired to do anything else. We took a taxi and returned to Jo's apartment, where Ross collapsed on a big leather sofa. He listened to music on the stereo and watched the Washington news on television.

"This sure is a nice place, Mom. What do you suppose it costs?"

"I have no idea. The rent is pretty high in this area."

"I'd like to have a place like this when I move to Washington," he said.

The next morning, Ross took a taxi to the metro station and returned to NIH, where he visited with the little boy who faced amputation of his leg. By the time he returned to Arlington, I had our bags packed. We went by taxi to National Airport.

Bill and Mary met us in Mobile when we arrived at 10:00 p.m. Mary hugged and kissed Ross, and Bill put his arm around his shoulder and said, "Welcome home, son. I know you're glad it's over."

"It's not over, Dad. I guess it will never be over."

∾

When I came home from work on Monday, he said, "Let's go up to the deli and get a big mushroom hamburger."

"Sure. When do you want to go?"

"Can we go now? I'm starved!"

Driving the short distance to the cafe, I remembered that we had not stayed in a hotel, and had eaten not a single meal in a restaurant on this last trip—a first in seven years.

Many times I had been invited to stay in someone's home in the vicinity of Bethesda, but couldn't accept the offer. In addition to the strange schedule I kept—coming and going at all hours of the night—in order to survive and try to keep my sanity, I had to be completely alone at times. My time away from the hospital was my chance to cry. If I gained nothing else from these experiences, I did learn that I have the right to choose my time and place to cry.

It was October 30, 1989, more than seven years from the diagnosis of osteosarcoma in Ross's left arm, and 16 months since the discovery of the same type tumor in his right leg.

At the deli, Ross and I sat outside in the chilled air as the traffic sped by on the other side of a thin wooden privacy wall. He'd had little to say on the plane home from Washington or throughout the weekend, but this evening he seemed to want to talk. I had seen him looking at want ads in the newspaper and I asked, "Are you looking for a job or a place to live?"

"Both...maybe. Or maybe neither. I do want to move out of the house as soon as I feel better, but I've got to have a job first. I'd like to wait until my hair comes back and I get over the treatment before I go on interviews."

"If you move out of the house, does it mean that I'll finally have a 'cat-free' existence?"

"No, the cats have to stay. It's their home."

"One of the first things I want you to do when you feel better is to go through all your newspapers and magazines. I can't clean the den for all your junk and college catalogues."

His only use of the computer had been to write to about 30

314 The Best I Can

colleges for information on their graduate school programs. But when the catalogues arrived, he never felt like studying them.

He spoke again of graduate school, still insisting that he would finance it himself. "Do you think Mr. Callahan could help me find a job in Washington?"

"I'm sure he'd be glad to try, Ross. You've got a good-looking resume. You need to go up there and pound the pavement like everybody else."

"Maybe if I could get a job in Washington, I could work on my masters at one of the universities there if they would accept me. Or I could get a job here and save money to get started. I'll have to wait until after the CT scan, though. And I still have the Port-A-Cath. I hope it can be removed soon so I can start physical therapy."

"Can you begin to think about trying to put all this behind you now and getting on with your life?" I asked.

"I guess so, as soon as I have the CT."

"I'm not worried about the CT, Ross. Try to put it out of your mind."

"It's not easy to do, you know."

"I know. But all that's going to happen next month is that they're going to tell you to come back again in another month, and on and on."

"Dr. Horowitz spends a lot of time in Africa. The next time I go up, I'm going to ask him if he knows of any program or job I might get where I could go along and assist in some way."

EPILOGUE

October, 1989—June, 1997

In April, 1990, six months after Ross finished chemotherapy treatments, he left for Prague, where he taught conversational English to students and faculty at the Czechoslovak Technical University. He volunteered for a four-month assignment through Education for Democracy/USA, Inc., which was founded in Mobile in February, 1990, about the time he had recuperated enough to get on with his life.

He became captivated by the concept of EFD/USA, and more than charmed by its founder and director, Ann Gardner. The grassroots program offered person-to-person assistance in learning to communicate in English, and was designed for the citizens of Czechoslovakia shortly after they staged their "velvet revolution" and escaped communist rule. Dr. Paul Demes, a physician from Bratislava who had studied at the University of South Alabama in Mobile, also had a position with the new government. Through his friendship with Ann Gardner and her husband, Dr. Bill Gardner, he inspired the concept of EFD/USA.

Ross left New York on Lufthansa Airlines and flew to Frankfurt, Germany, then on to Prague, where he was met by a Czechoslovakian girl who spoke no English. She delivered him to EFD/USA's field office, where the staff helped him find the house of the family with whom he would be living.

He telephoned home twice, but there was so much to tell that he gave up, promising to write. His busy schedule kept him occupied, but we finally received his five-page letter written on a day he had to stay in because he was ill with a virus. He wrote of the "tasty"cabbage and potatoes he ate almost every day, and of his host family—a husband, wife, and two children who spoke little English and practiced with him whenever possible. He walked a mile each morning to catch a bus, which he rode for thirty minutes before switching to a train. When he got off the train, he had another mile-long hike to the university where he taught.

In one of his telephone calls home, he said he was astounded at the misconceptions the students had about our country, but impressed by their academic abilities and how far beyond us they had advanced in other areas. After classes, he ran around with the students and stayed late in the evenings at coffee houses and theaters. His days began at 7:00 a.m. and ended at midnight.

He had to make one hurried trip back home at the end of May for a CT scan, and since he was a little homesick, he opted to come to Mobile for it instead of going to NIH. The scan results were shipped to NIH, and in three days, he returned to Prague, where he moved into a college dorm.

During his remaining two months in Europe, he went by train with a student to his home in a little village near Wroclaw, Poland. Later, he rode with students in an old Skoda to East Germany where he visited the site of the infamous Berlin wall. After several days in Germany, they left for Prague, and Ross took a turn at the wheel while on the autobahn.

When his assignment ended in July, he returned to Mobile, then went to NIH for a check-up. Three suspicious nodules were found in his lungs. He would have to be rechecked monthly.

A thoracotomy was performed in October, 1990, and five nodules were removed. Three of them tested positive for malignancy.

After six weeks of recuperation from the surgery, he traveled with Ann Gardner to the Slovak region for a conference on volunteerism which was held in a castle somewhere near Bratislava. Ross came home with a special Christmas gift—a letter from President Vaclav Havel—thanking him for his service.

At home, Ross was deeply involved with his activities, but he was not too busy to see the beginning of the end of his parents' marriage. Bill and I separated in April, 1991. Bill moved first to Troy to be with his mother, who was very ill, then relocated to Birmingham where he continued practicing architecture.

Ross had taken a part-time job at Spring Hill College so he could devote time and energy to EFD/USA, Inc. at their head-quarters office in Mobile. The program had attracted nationwide attention through coverage in *The Washington Post* and *The New York Times,* as well as some foreign publications. Their makeshift borrowed office swelled with applications from those who want-ed to volunteer, and from organizations in Czechoslovakia who wanted them to come. Placement, travel arrangements, housing, logistics, and coordination kept the phones ringing and the fax machine humming. Our home telephone number got into the sys-tem, and calls came from all over during the day and night.

During Ross's hectic schedule, he took breaks to go for check-ups at NIH. His CT scans remained clear until October, 1991, when two spots appeared. Another thoracotomy was done on December 9th, and three nodules were removed, all of them malignant.

While Ross recuperated at home from the surgery, he threw himself back into the exciting work of EFD/USA, Inc. He set up their fax machine on our kitchen counter and labored over grant-proposals at the computer.

He took the GRE exam, applied to graduate schools, and in March, 1992, he received his acceptance from American University in Washington. He was to enter for the fall semester.

In April, his CT scan revealed still another spot which would have to be checked each month.

While watching and waiting, he decided, painfully, to give up his work with EFD/USA, Inc., in order to take a course at the Institute of World Politics, which began in May in Washington. The course proved to be one of the most rewarding academic endeavors he had ever experienced, and it stimulated him even more to pursue his goal of a career in international studies. While there, he rented a college dorm room near the Institute and scouted around for a place to live when he began classes at American University.

His third thoracotomy was performed on July 14, 1992. Before he was admitted to the hospital, he drove me to American University to show me the campus and the neighborhood. We stopped for lunch at the Hamburger Hamlet on Wisconsin Avenue.

After recuperating at home in Mobile, he returned to Washington and began classes the end of August. He moved into a house in Chevy Chase, which he shared with James Hutchins, whose travels around the world had landed him there. Sabin Bokus, another Spring Hill College friend who was now in graduate school at American, moved in with them.

Ross wrote volumes of research papers, attended lectures at other colleges, spent hours in the library, studied hard, and made good grades and new friends. He and his housemates had dinner parties and kept open house for visitors who needed a place to stay for a few days.

He spent Christmas in Mobile and New Year's in New Orleans with Natalie. Her work with an organization which served the poverty-stricken inner city people had carried her to England and France, but had also brought her to Louisiana.

After beginning classes again at American University the first week in January, 1993, he returned to NIH to learn that yet another spot had been found in a lung. It had to be watched with monthly scans. In February, the spot had grown "explosively" and, more importantly, another foreboding spot was discovered between his lungs in the center of his chest, near his heart.

Dr. Horowitz was on sabbatical, and Dr. Leonard Wexler, a former Clinical Associate, had been appointed to his position. When Ross met in conference with Dr. Wexler, Ann Marie Gamble, a former classmate from Spring Hill College, went with him.

Ann Marie called me in Mobile after the conference. She said that Dr. Wexler told Ross that consultation with Dr. Pass, the thoracic surgeon, indicated the spot between his lungs appeared to be inoperable. He encouraged Ross to take the only other option—chemotherapy. At first, Ross said, "No," but later, he agreed to consider it.

The next day, Sabin drove Ross on a wild and flying trip to New Orleans for Mardi Gras where they stayed with Natalie. She joined forces with James, Sabin, Ann Marie, and other friends in talking Ross into accepting the treatment, assuring him they would stand by and support him all the way.

Sabin and Ross drove all day and all night from New Orleans in order to keep his appointment at NIH. Ross had just arrived back in Maryland when he met me in the clinic. Tired and bleary-eyed, he avoided looking me in the eyes when he and Dr. Wexler came into the waiting room. He hugged me tightly, then quickly left the room.

Dr. Wexler, a curly-haired young man with a face full of beard and smile, wore a yarmulke. As he sat in a chair beside me, he spoke about Ross's new developments, and he withheld no truths. He assured me he would not recommend that Ross go through chemotherapy again unless he believed there was a chance that it could destroy the cancer cells. He had consulted with others at NIH and throughout the country, and with Dr. Horowitz. Everyone agreed: It was worth a try.

The plan was to schedule treatments of VP 16 along with Ifosphamide. VP 16 was the drug which had been removed from Ross's protocol in 1989. As before, it would be given five days in a row, every three weeks.

He began the treatment on Friday, and on Sunday, I invited James, Ann Marie, and Sabin to breakfast at the Marriott. Sabin brought his pretty blonde girlfriend from Germany, Sabena, who was on an extended visit at the house in Chevy Chase.

When they arrived in the lobby, they were dressed in heavy coats, boots, caps, and mufflers. During greetings and introductions, they each hugged me tightly.

Ann Marie, tall and willowy, with fair skin and dark brown eyes, had her long dark auburn hair up in a bun, enhancing her graceful sophistication and classic beauty.

James was in Washington scouting around for opportunities in social work while maintaining two part-time jobs. His blue eyes had deepened in color. Two years of working with "Fourth

World" masses in inner cities had carved a deep well of caring and compassion.

Sabin, cosmopolitan and demonstrative, kept his French beret on after he removed his black trench coat. Sabena worked for a news agency in Berlin and was on assignment in Washington.

After we finished breakfast in Allie's Pantry, all five of us went to my room. Ross's friends sat on the bed and the floor and listened while I tried to tell them what to expect if they were going to be his caregivers. Ann Marie would take on the task of locating and helping prepare foods Ross might eat. James and Sabin would run the errands and do the chauffeuring. Sabena would act as nurse-in-residence for the time she was there.

Ross's symptoms after the first series of treatments were the same as all his sessions in years past. Three weeks later, before the second round of chemotherapy, he had a Port-A-Cath put in place again since his previous one had been removed before he left for Prague in 1990. After discharge from the hospital, while back at the house in Chevy Chase, he suffered a fever and had to be admitted to the hospital for IV antibiotics. Then, a few days after being discharged, his red blood count dropped. Again, he had to be hospitalized for a transfusion of packed red cells.

With the help of his friends, Ross tried the third round of treatment as an outpatient. But there were too many trips back and forth to the hospital for various problems, fevers, and blood transfusions. He sorrowfully admitted that he couldn't remain in school, and would have to move back to Mobile to continue his treatment at the Mobile Infirmary.

He arranged with American University to take an "incomplete"on his college work and would try to finish his papers while at home. James helped him pack and store his things.

Ross asked Dr. Wexler for a 10-day postponement of the fourth round of treatment in Mobile in order to accept Ann Gardner's invitation to accompany her to Bratislava. He and Ann met at JFK Airport in New York, where they drank a champagne toast before boarding Austrian Airlines and flying to Vienna. They were met by a car and driver and taken to Bratislava, which was now in its own country, Slovakia. Upon arrival, they attended a reception.

The next day, they went by bus for an overnight trip to Prague, so Ross could visit his friends there.

When they got back to Bratislava, Ross's strength was depleted and he had to remain in bed while Ann continued her appointments throughout the Slovak region. Later in the week, he recuperated enough to join her.

They returned to Mobile late Monday night, and on Wednesday Ross saw Dr. Clarkson and continued treatment at the Mobile Infirmary. Transfusions of red blood cells in increasing amounts combined with high fevers kept sending him back to the hospital between treatments. When at home, he gave himself a daily injection of a drug to help bring his white blood count up from critical levels.

In addition to losing all of his hair, eyebrows, and eyelashes for the fourth time, he also quickly lost 35 pounds.

A few days after he had finished the seventh round of treatment on August 2, 1993, he was admitted to the emergency room for a transfusion of platelets and packed red blood cells.

While in the hospital bed, hooked up to the IV, he tearfully tried to tell Dr. Clarkson that he couldn't continue treatment. I tightened my lips and covered them with my fingers as I listened. When he could no longer speak, I tried to finish his thoughts. Instead, I, too, wept.

Dr. Clarkson looked from Ross to me, but said nothing. He picked up Ross's record and quickly wrote, "Battle fatigue. Discharge."

After being released from the hospital the next day, Ross wrote and faxed a letter to Dr. Wexler:

> "...I am physically and mentally very tired, and every treatment I've had so far seems to bring me down in both respects more and more each time...I have to tell you honestly that I would like to stop them now...Over the past few weeks my will to continue has diminished greatly and I'm afraid of pushing myself beyond what I think my capacity for tolerance and endurance will allow.
>
> "Dr. Raj told me about the possibility of a surgical

option when he called me last week and I am very interested in exploring this...I understand that the metastases inside and outside my lungs are 'stable,' meaning no growth, which seems to be indicated by my most recent scans. I understand as well that they are 'calcified' and, that being the fact, the spots on the X-rays may never disappear on film, and they may not even shrink any more than they already have. I suppose it follows then that the only way to verify whether or not the tumors are dying or are dead is to have them removed.

"Are you (or Dr. Pass) willing to consider surgery now because the tumors do not appear to be shrinking after seven treatments? Do you think they might shrink more if I continued...? When I began this treatment, Dr. Pass had indicated that surgery was not an option at that time. What has changed since then to make it more of a possibility?...Or, is this offer for a possible surgery simply a shot in the dark...and an attempt to address my wish to stop chemotherapy...?

"Dr. Wexler,...I want to know if you still maintain the same level of optimism about the treatments' effectiveness that you had when I began the treatments in February. Do you still believe a cure is possible, or is that contingent on my completing twelve cycles? Or is it contingent on twelve cycles and surgery?

"Do you have any new or different therapies that I might be able to try? You mentioned something to me about some sort of growth hormone inhibitor...Is that a possibility? Also, I asked you about the macrophage agent...that I learned about from M. D. Anderson in Houston. Could this be a possibility? I must tell you, however, that any new chemotherapy or other drug therapy that I might be able to consider would have to be much more easily tolerated physically than the current treatments have been. If there would be similar side effects...then I can't imagine that they would have any less negative effects on me physically or mentally, and I would be in the same dilemma that I find myself now....

"...I very much need your reassurance and confidence concerning my condition and the prospects for my future. Without your reassurance, it becomes more difficult for me to maintain my will to continue this fight...."

After he sent the letter to Dr. Wexler, he visited Dr. Clarkson to finish what he had tried to say while in the hospital. He expressed the same thoughts and questions to him as he did in his letter to Dr. Wexler. He talked about his beliefs and feelings concerning quality versus quantity of life.

Soon after he made his decision, he and I spent the weekend at the Mullers' house at Gulf Shores. It was his 29th birthday, and he found the strength to walk out on piers and around marinas to look at sailboats and dream of a life of ease.

Dr. Pass and other surgeons looked again at the X-rays and tentatively decided to do the risky surgery on September 28, 1993. However, after Ross's pulmonary function tests revealed that his breathing capacity had deteriorated, and his generally debilitated condition had not improved, the doctors changed their minds. Under the most ideal circumstances, the surgery would be dangerous. Getting to the growth in the middle of his chest would require removal of the entire right lung with no assurance that all of the nodule could be excised. He would be oxygen-dependent for the rest of his life. They had to tell Ross that he might not survive the operation.

Bill and I were in the waiting room while Ross was in conference with the surgeons. When Ross joined us, he sat down, bent forward with his elbow resting on his knee, and covered his eyes with his hand.

But soon he pulled himself together and left for the metro to go to American University and visit a professor with whom he had established a close personal relationship. When he returned to the Marriott that evening, he made plans for us to go out to dinner. He telephoned Bill at his hotel and asked him to meet us at the Medical Center metro station. We rode the metro to Chevy

Chase and had dinner in one of his favorite restaurants on Wisconsin Avenue. He acted as our escort, ushering us from place to place, telling us where to sit, and what to order from the menu. All of us left to return to Alabama the next day—Ross and I to Mobile, and Bill to Birmingham where he had lived since our divorce in June, 1991.

Again, a month later, when Ross's physical condition had improved marginally, he met with surgeons after a CT scan and pulmonary function tests. The scans indicated that the spot in his lung tissue had shrunk dramatically, and both spots showed dense calcification, but the surgical prognosis was still the same. This time, Ross made the decision that he would not have the operation.

The break-up of their parents left a permanent scar on all our children. It would be four years before Bill and I could establish any communication and cautiously investigate the possibility of a reconciliation.

Other major events affected all our lives during that time. The month before he left on his first trip to Prague in April, 1990, Ross had delivered the eulogy at his Aunt Dorothy Riorda's funeral in New Orleans. She died less than three months after having been diagnosed with metastatic lung cancer. His Aunt Hilda Heflin in California had lost her battle with non-Hodgkins lymphoma in June, 1991, less than three years after it was discovered.

After living at home for more than a year, Mary learned that her heart was still in Virginia. She returned there and accepted a job with United Airlines. When Scott decided to return to Mobile from Huntsville, he entered the University of South Alabama, where he buckled down and often made the Dean's List. After graduation, he remained at home and worked for a year, then left for graduate school at North Carolina State University in Raleigh. Later, he postponed graduate studies in order to accept a job with the Town of Smithfield, near Raleigh, as a Geographical Information Systems specialist.

Ross spent his recuperating months in Mobile, with occasional trips to Birmingham to visit his dad. He went to New Orleans for Mardi Gras in February, 1994, with several American

University friends who had driven down. Slowly, his weight, color, and energy returned. Most of his hair did not return.

He visited my weekly writing group, decided to join us, and produced a poignant story, "Best Friends," which was accepted for publication in the anthology *Home Again, Home Again.* He spent hours working on his new notebook computer while listening to his favorite music.

While writing and keeping up with events in Europe through television and the periodicals that came to him, he took time out to play with Maggie, Mitty, Mikey, and our black lab, Pepper. Three goldfish survived in the overgrown and neglected pond.

In May, 1994, Ross, Mary, and I flew to Prague where we stayed for the first week of our vacation. Mary acted as our travel agent, but Ross was tour-guide, proudly showing us the city he had learned to love. After Mary returned to Virginia, Ross and I remained in Prague for a few days, then went by bus to Vienna, by boat on the Danube to Budapest, by train to Bratislava, then back to Prague before returning to Mobile. Although Ross's stamina was still limited, I soon learned it surpassed my own. My heavy backpack and hiking boots on cobblestone streets, rushing to catch city buses and underground trains, and late nights in coffeehouses and pubs took their toll.

But it was all that was needed to rekindle Ross's interest in pursuing his studies in international affairs. He returned to American University in August, 1994.

Luckily, some of his former housemates had room for him in their new place in Arlington, Virginia. The household had many visitors for overnights, weekends, or longer. The permanent residents changed from time to time. James had left Washington, but returned after getting his graduate degree from Auburn University; Josh was there when Ross moved in but went to India for several months, then returned. Jed, Ellen, Dan, and the household pet, a big Walker hound named Blue, made up the rest of the long-time residents.

With Ross settled, I began to turn my thoughts to my own life. Ross's advice to me back in 1988 haunted me: *"Stop putting off things you want to do with your life."* I remembered my two sisters,

Dorothy and Hilda. Like most everyone else, both of them had thought they had many years yet to live.

In June, 1995, I made a major decision and resigned my stressful job as district office manager for the First Congressional District of Alabama. The loyal support I had received from Congressman Callahan and his staff would continue.

When Ross first arrived back in Washington in August, 1994, he went to NIH for tests and scans. The nodules were still there, unchanged. Dr. Wexler told him that since there had been no change for more than a year, he was again considered to be in remission. In 1995, and again in 1996, he received the same report.

After a particularly strenuous hiking and camping trip in 1996, his right leg began hurting. Tests and X-rays revealed a problem with the internal prosthesis in his leg. Although it had been anticipated the prosthesis would last for 12 years when it was implanted in 1988, the X-ray revealed that repairs were necessary.

Ross hoped to postpone the surgery until he finished his graduate studies and research papers; however, after limping around in pain for several months, and being unable to go wherever he wanted, he found it impossible to delay the operation.

On May 27, 1997, Bill and I met him at 5:00 a.m. at the Washington Hospital Center when Jed, one of his housemates, drove him there. We sat on either side him in the admitting office while waiting for an attendant to come and escort him to surgery. He was very quiet, and I knew he was psyching himself up for surgery, as he had always done in the past.

After the surgery was finished, Dr. Martin Malawer came out to the waiting room to talk to Bill and me. He explained that the end of the bone of the femur, where the original implant had been placed, had become porous and brittle, resulting in loss of stability. He removed two more inches of the femur and put a new prosthesis there. Part of the knee portion of the implant had broken or become loosened, and that was replaced and repaired. The tibia portion of the original implant was in excellent condition.

Then Dr. Malawer smiled and quickly added, "I saw no sign of tumor anywhere in his leg." He was very pleased with how well the surgery went, and said that although he had planned a four-hour procedure, it had taken only two hours. He told us that

Ross's leg should be in better shape now than it had been almost nine years ago when he did the first surgery.

When Ross was returned to his room, he was hooked up to all kinds of tubes and wires. A catheter was in place in the carotid artery in his neck. He was in intense pain, and Bill and I took turns spending the night with him.

After a few days, Bill returned to Birmingham, and I planned to remain with Ross until he was discharged from the hospital and got his strength back.

Once the pain was under control, and he was unhooked from some of the confining tubes, Ross made a remarkably quick recovery. He sat up in bed smiling and chatting with his many visitors. Seven days after surgery, he began practicing walking on crutches. On the eighth day, when Dr. Malawer and his associates visited him to see if he was ready for discharge, Dr. Malawer asked him to stand by the bed. Ross complied, putting weight on his right leg. Then Dr. Malawer told him to try walking. Ross reached for his crutches, but Dr. Malawer held up his hand and said, "Try it without the crutches."

Ross looked at the doctor, questioning. Then he took a deep breath, straightened his shoulders, and walked a few steps. With a big smile, he reached out and shook hands with Dr. Malawer.

Later that day, while the social worker was making her daily visit, she asked Ross to visit another patient on the hall. A man in his forties had been diagnosed with osteosarcoma in his leg and was scheduled for surgery by Dr. Malawer.

While Ross bathed and dressed for the visit, I sat in a lounge at the end of the hall. In a little while, I saw him coming out of his room on crutches. He slowly walked along the hall and went into the man's room near the nurse's station. As I watched him, an apt, descriptive expression I had read and heard came to mind: "Wounded healer."

Ross's clothes had been packed, so while I waited for him, I went to the first floor and out into the courtyard of the massive, sprawling hospital complex. May had slipped into June, and, although the sun was shining, it was unseasonably cool. I shivered under my light-weight cotton sweater.

I sat at a wrought iron table under an arbor covered with

wisteria vines and remembered that I needed to call Bill, Mary, and Scott to let them know Ross was being discharged. With the support of his housemates and many friends, he wouldn't need me for more than a week, and I could return home to Mobile.

Thinking of home, I wondered what might be going on there that needed my attention. I thought of the pets and hoped the staff of the kennel where Pepper was boarded were giving her attention and affection. I wondered how many more times I could call on my brother-in-law, Joe Croom, to feed the cats and water my plants. I thought of the Mahonys next door who always kept a watchful eye on my house and collected my mail and newspapers.

There would be no way to ever repay all the people who had helped us. The faces of all those who continued to pray and give moral support for almost fifteen years came to mind. No, it's never possible to repay anyone, I thought, but we can pass it on to another who needs it. We can do the best we can.

In the courtyard, I looked up at the third-floor window to Ross's room and saw him standing there looking down at me. He held up his hand and waved to me, giving the victory sign—it was time to leave. His friend Chris had arrived to haul us to Arlington in his station wagon.

With a lightened heart, I breathed a grateful sigh as a contentment moved within me. I smiled when I rose from my chair, waved back to Ross, and remembered an expression I had heard my pastor, Vernon Hunter, say recently: "Kiss the joys as they fly by."